The
Three
Treasures

Other Books By Tina Chunna Zhang

Classical Northern Wu Style Tai Ji Quan:
   The Fighting Art of the Manchurian Palace Guard (with Frank Allen)

The Whirling Circles of Ba Gua Zhang:
   The Art and Legends of the Eight Trigram Palm (with Frank Allen)

Earth Qi Gong for Women:
   Awaken Your Inner Healing Power

The Three Treasures

Traditional Chinese Medical Qi Gong for Health

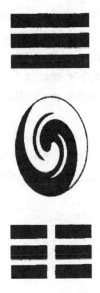

Tina Chunna Zhang

Copy right © 2012 by Tina Chunna Zhang. All rights reserved. No portion of this book may be reproduced, stored in retrieval system, or transmitted in any form or by any means - electronic, mechanical, photocopying, recording, or otherwise - without written permission of the author.

PLEASE NOTE: The creator of this book is not and will not be responsible in any way whatsoever, for any improper use made by anyone of the information contained in this book. All use of the aforementioned information must be made in accordance with what is permitted by law, and any damage liable to be caused as result thereof will be the exclusive responsibility of the user. in addition, he or she must adhere strictly to the safety rules contained in the book, both in training and in actual implementation of the information presented herein. This book is intended for use in conjunction with ongoing lessons and personal training with an authorized expert. The instructions and advice printed in this book are not in any way intended as a substitute for medical mental, or emotional counseling with a licensed physician or healthcare provider.

Summary: Focuses on promoting health through Traditional Chinese Medicine method and ancient Chinese Taoist philosophy through series of gentle, conscious Qi Gong movement to achieve a healthy living.

© 2012 Lulu Author. All rights reserved.
   ISBN 978-1-105-66368-0
   Content ID: 12792672
   Book title: The Three Treasures

Contents

Foreword

Preventive health care has these days finally received the attention it deserves.

As we age, the gradual failure of organs, sometimes including the marrow and the brain can present a challenge that is often beyond the reach of the most assiduous of physicians.

The benefits of diet, exercise and the reduction of self administered toxins are in western medical terms well supported with evidence, the most recent of which clearly shows gains in longevity and reduction in cancer rates in those who exercise regularly. Sadly for many, these types of lifestyle changes are too difficult, yet reliance on medicines has become common.

The technologies of western medicine have produced many benefits but not as yet effective anti-aging methods, though the search goes on. Early Taoists reportedly often poisoned themselves and others while searching for an "elixir of life." Later it was finally realized that the true answers lay within. Nearly a thousand years later, western physicians were also administrating poisons such as arsenicals to their patients, at a time when the West was first introduced to what we now recognize as Qigong, though the works of Père Amiot (1718-1793) and Dudgeon (1895).

These days the well intentioned efforts of physicians may unfortunately, still result in excessive and inappropriate prescribing.

Far better then for us, in as far as we are able, to take some personal responsibility and to try to preserve our own health.

Breathing, meditation and similar practices have never been a preoccupation of western medicine, although certainly Galen and Oribasius described four types of breathing. Awareness of such techniques in recent times probably began for many with the emerging popularity of yoga in the 1930s.

In this book Tina Zhang introduces what is needed to succeed and guides us through the language of Chinese medicine.

Research in Qi Gong and meditation has sadly lagged behind that of exercise. New research findings in neuropsychology or neurobiology regarding these may eventually reveal some mechanisms, (whether it be hormonal release, altered telomerase levels, neuroplasticity and morphology or something unexpected). While this is interesting, it is not necessarily important to those who find benefit from practicing these techniques.

In order to benefit fully one needs perseverance but also guidance from a high level practitioner with a sound appreciation of their subject. Qi Gong and similar activities can often lend themselves to excessive theorising. Tina Zhang however, as well as being able to explain the theoretical base, can also call on a lifetime of practical application of these principals, the seemingly magical combination of inner activity, Nei Gong with (external) strengthening, Qiang Zhuang Gong that is found necessary to nourish life.

Dr. Jon Lismore
England

Preface

Heaven has three treasures – The Sun, The Moon, and The Stars.
Earth possesses three treasures – Water, Fire, and Wind.
Human beings create three treasures – Essence, Energy, and Spirit.
Wise applications of these three treasures liberate us to eternity.

"Dao gives the birth to one; one gives the birth to two; two gives the birth to three; three gives birth to everything; when do all things awaken?" - Dao De Jing

The Three Treasures is the title of an ancient Chinese philosophy that acknowledges the relationships between Heaven, Earth, and human beings. The greatest benefits of Qi Gong for health come from the treasures of Traditional Chinese Medicine, Taoist philosophy, and Internal Martial Arts.

Medical Qi Gong is an ancient Chinese health exercise based on the theories of Traditional Chinese Medicine that focus on the human body's internal energy balance; and it's about working with your own energy to have better health. The Chinese body-mind-spirit ideal of health is best achieved when human beings in perfect resonance with nature at one unified circle.

This set of medical Qi Gong exercises was created by long time study, diligent research and by an understanding the grace of Daoist culture. There is a classical sayings in Chinese: "从医入道，道以医显，Studying medicine is entering the Dao; the Dao always appears within the medicine." As a life long internal martial artist, Qi Gong and Traditional Chinese Medicine practitioner, blending the knowledge of these traditions, I proudly reformed their magical existence and explain in details the correlation to the theory of Chinese medicine. Using the Qi Gong as a prat of clinical treatment during my years of practice, I have seen so many people changed from the fatigue and pain to positively improved of various health conditions. It's a joy to see this classical health art to be preserved, introduced to more people on the Earth!

The meridian theory and its relationship to Qi Gong practice for health is the topic of this book, not other theories of Traditional Chinese Medicine will be discussed.

The style of writing of this book is designed in approaching for an easy reading and, an accessible way to understand Chinese philosophy, traditional medicine and Qi Gong practice.

The Chinese language used in this book is the Pin Yin system, for example: "Tai Chi," will be written as Tai Ji Quan. Hopefully, some Chinese characters in the book will be understood straightly for people who know Chinese language.

This book is dedicated to people who love extraordinary health.

Tina Chunna Zhang

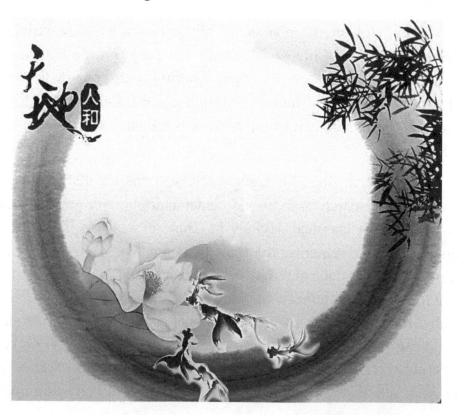

Introduction

Medical Qi Gong is a branch of ancient Chinese energetic and a healing system of Traditional Chinese Medicine that we are practicing in China; along with acupuncture, herbal medicine, and Tui Na, to nurtures life and keep healthy. The goal of medical Qi Gong is to correct these bio-energetic imbalance and blockages which believed as the cause of all illnesses. We practice these particular Qi Gong form exercise and meditation to strengthen and regulate the functions of internal organs and systems. The medical Qi Gong practice enables human body and the mind waking up and gaining the power to relieve pains in physical and deep-seated emotions; the medical Qi Gong treatment serves as preventive health care as well as complementary and alternative medicine!

The medical Qi Gong in this book is combination of classic Qi Gong with new research and development of Traditional Chinese Medicine in China.

Since ancient time, Dr. Hou Tuo, the Father of Traditional Chinese Medicine invented Five Animal Frolics to use certain movements as energy medicine for people to keep good health and to heal, there are many Chinese Traditional Medicine doctors and martial arts masters devoted their life time to further the development and refinement to this wonderful healing art through generations.

The Three Treasures medical Qi Gong and Traditional Chinese Medicine has an inner connection, they share classical philosophy and methodology based on and guided by the theory of the meridians, they have the similar purpose. The beauty of the medical Qi Gong is that can be naturally and particularly serves as self-energy cultivation exercise to achieve desired result, and a practical way to understand the meridians of human body and working with body's energy points and channels.

The Three Treasures Medical Qi Gong integrates the classical Chinese concept of the harmony of the three treasures of the Heaven, Earth, and Human into Qi Gong practice, and it breaks through with its special touches and emphasizes on these well established fourteen meridian channels Qi flow, which nurturing and cultivating the energy of the body.

As Tina Zhang addressed: "The Three Treasures medical Qi Gong promotes health through deep breathing, gentle motion, and relaxed intention." The Three Treasures medical Qi Gong is an easy to learn and manageable for self-practice, and doable for anyone in any ages and physical conditions, with or without Chinese medicine knowledge.

Healthy and happy to all!

Dr. Xu Zhi Min
Traditional Chinese Medicine
Beijing, China

Chapter 1

Values of Ancient Qi Gong for a Modern Living

Powering the Mind

"When Heaven is about to place a responsibility on a great human, it always first frustrates his spirit and will, toughen his nature and enhance his abilities." - Lao Zi

We are living in a fantastic world, with so many advanced technologies, and we come to expect something new to enter our lives everyday that wonderfully serves our needs and adds to our convenience, as well as our fast pace of life. Many things we used to do with, things we owned dearly, seems to have faded out, or been replaced quickly by something new and fancy. In our current lives, we fantasize about generations of Chinese Emperors, and Western Kings who could never even dreamed of luxury life. Each day, some things and thoughts exists less and less of the old ways of living. The mind changes the world!

Since the only constant in the universe is developing and change, all matters can only exist for as long as their ultimate nature as pure potential is resisted. Human's mind has power that believes, creates, and controls the activities. We are familiar with the fact that the air travel system today came from a belief; the organ replacement to save a life is due to its initial thought of the possibility. Everything in creation occurred first as an awareness of what was possible, then, intentional actions made it a reality. In ancient Chinese belief, Qi, human life force energy, made everything possible, and the Qi of the creativity is putting oneself beyond possibilities, to achieve the "impossibilities."

In the world we are lucky to be living is great, and we have been experiencing so much joy and definitely hope to gracefully live longer. We all acknowledge that this is not any more of the world where people simply work for gaining the basic conditions of life - food and shelter. We are living in human being's healthiest time with our best overall longevity rate. This fact has become an integral part of our personal identity and evolutionary journey, that leads to a natural retuning journey to the original birth. We need to have a mind that thinking, it is possible to live a long and sickness free life. This belief makes the dream, the dream makes us think, thinking creates the action, the action results the possibilities!

However, just providing yourself a life with new technology and a good environment does not mean that you have achieved a fulfilled life in today's world. A human's life achievement and enjoyment is far beyond only satisfying the current surroundings and technologies. It is its unlimited potential that is continuously expressed by more powerful creativity that serves better livings - this all comes from our minds - the power house.

The mind set on something to achieve in our life time is a challenge, especially, if it's not constructed from scientifically approved matters and activities. Such as the case of a superior Chinese health exercise called Qi Gong, which came from ancient times and beliefs. It remains in its own right, as well as mystery. Therefore, Qi Gong is not a common ground with the discoveries by modern science that can proof a human being's deeper mental and physical potentials. We hope that someday science can find answers for the curious things that have no answers today, so the old alchemy can truly meet science. Meanwhile, so many minds in this world are believing in Qi Gong and Tai Ji Quan, and practice these arts for promoting the general health. Positive results have been recently reported to the public from both the eastern and western medical fields!

It is a strong belief that one should set up a path worth traveling. Whether the Chinese concept of Qi has been proved by science or not, it's worth to continue the art that came from a long history. Therefore, the art of Qi, has been culturally and practically established, accepted, and practiced by so many people. Qi, as vital energy lays inside the body and mind, through the Qi Gong exercise, many bodies become healthier. Especially, the mind can be powered by the flow of the Qi, too! Qi is not something gained through the sense of the external organs, it's the connections and feelings from inner oneself. This is because inner activity changes, dominates, and balances the thoughts and actions of a human being. Therefore, these profound Qi Gong exercises coupled with Daoist philosophy become a balanced action as a revolution into this fantasy yet reality world, which is not only limited to the physical improvement, but to challenges the mind.

The minds needs power to take challenges to enable them to go further. The mind needs exercise to stay sharp; the mind also needs rest and relax like all parts of the body. Facing a world with a very fast-paced daily life, the mind, with its extremely busy way of following matters, sudden changes can cause the mind to be overwhelmed, and lose its focus, the eyes that are behind the mind are blurry and cannot see the future picture clearly – through this stress is created, which causes the mind to be unable to fully function on its own potentials. Some people collapse on the road of experiencing life, their minds do not have enough power to deal with reality, and their health are declines. The fulfillments of life get away from them, no matter how much high tech and extensive supplies are provided for them, their minds drag their bodies away from truly being alive.

The power of the mind comes out of calmness and awareness, the grounding of the mind should be solid and stable, which is also the base for focus and creativity. Qi Gong, is mind training within highly involved exercises, that differ from exercises based on only gaining muscle; Qi Gong exercise is coordinated through physical motion to build a new relationship between the body and mind through slow but focused actions. Slow motion in Qi Gong really gives the time that the mind and body need for sensing, relaxing, and focusing. As the intension is increased slowly, that helps to achieve harmony of the mind and body. A calmness based sensation will be developed, which help awareness, imagination and creativity, that help the mind free from darkness in order to realize whatever is life's enjoyment or desired purpose.

The mind balances and controls activities. Balance is the guide for everything, and control is the key to success. If you think too much sometime, decisions are never been made and opportunity is gone, but taking to fast and immature actions bring the same result. The regrets left to you can cause a pause in your smooth and continuous forward motion. Qi Gong exercises are intentional, yet natural exercises that train the mind with a Chinese Daoist philosophy based view of looking at life and the world, it balances the mind from too tight way of thinking.

Power of the Mind comes out of mental clearness.

The mind will have more power if it can be turned towards the inside to find the central point of stillness. Some people, seem never tired of seeking something new: new car, new house, new entertainment, new computer, new relationship, new things every day, happily owning them and temporarily pleased with their life, but not necessarily satisfied by what they have, because these things are just a reflection in their mind from their most outer existence. For the people who can turn their mind inward to look at their deep insides and their true image and reality, they can absorb what they learn and what they enjoyed lies stably inside their mind, instead of just a reflection in the mind. This looking inside of mind in Qi Gong exercises, will peel off the layers that block one looking within, so one can hold what he or she has dearly, perfectly, and long lasting, including relationships and materials.

All the methods we have acknowledged now are from ancient China. It took a long time to have them tested by generations of lives and become methods with new meaning to serve our present living. Don't you think this could be special value and worth to try?

Nurturing the Body

Yellow Emperor's Classic of Internal Medicine tells us: "Motion is to keep the body healthy; intention is to nurture the heart. Stillness is the root of cultivating the soul, and movement is the base in preserving health."

A healthy body is created by balanced energy.

Health, in traditional Chinese culture, is not only the treatment of illness or limited to not getting ill, but also a life long journey to discover your own body, observe your own habits, attitudes, and understand your own mind. Every posture or activity is either a health builder or health enemy; being healthy is a style of living.

Everything is changing in life, relatively, some things do not really change that much, or that fast such as our body shape. Thinking about this: when we are grown up and have attained our full size and strength in our adulthood we do not change much in this very short life. Even so, slow changes are happening throughout the different stages of life A mature body needs to keep in appropriate condition to support its natural growth and development, and only a completely healthy body can be a powerful system that can defeat our coming negativities. To live well, with brilliant ideas, creative mind, we need to eliminate physical problems, disorders, or any abnormal conditions; or whatever nightmares of unhealthy patterns that due to a person's genetic make up or the pollutants or any other external environment. To eliminate harm is to build a realistic healthy life style pattern that is more naturally based and continuously developed according to the universe and a human's prenatal energy.

As matter of a great fact, the world we live has been focused on the medical science and treatment to save life, to treat disease, and to make successful surgical! Meanwhile, do we ever try to bring our focus on prevention of diseases that harm our body's system first? Do we ever think that we can really achieve living an illness free life? Like all discovery that were made by the human mind, all of us can be profound thinkers and researchers to discover the true value of energy in our bodies that are already a natural strong system within itself, which builds natural functions to correct the dysfunctions.

Qi in Modern Times

Unlike the ancients, we now know that DNA is the blueprint for all the processes and structures of life. Genes are the basic functional units of heredity. Our health and illnesses all are related to DNA. But nothing is always in the same stage or condition when we grow older. The physical appearance and health condition are not only based upon the genetic codes, but are also affected and modified by many internal and external conditions. Especially, our health or illness that result from the interactions between the genes and living conditions. Even the shape of the body can be changed by body building or different kind of physical trainings. The body's internal environment is directly associated with our diet, lifestyle, daily activities, sleep quality, working condition, emotional and mental stress levels that determines one's health.

Qi cultivation is the core of Qi Gong practice which functions as a behavioral modifier to increase self-awareness our of levels of internal energy conditions. This helps us to contend with difficulties from stress and energy imbalance that occur during daily life. Through its gentle motions, it achieves an optimal state for our internal and external conditions which bring greater balance and harmony, and retrain the body for producing effective corresponding as "medicine" within itself, which will allow the body to heal.

In times long past, the old wisdom and experience of traditional Chinese medicine, that is heavily involved in nurturing life, served people's health in China. In some ways, a likeness of today's diet and exercise programs to keep healthy. The difference is that the Chinese way of exercise is always based on, or mixed with, or guided by philosophy and inner cultivation. The Chinese way of health is a way of life, and consists of the principles that apply to one's lifestyle.

Traditional Chinese Medicine is a culture based on philosophy. You cannot always completely translate one culture to another from the opposite world easily, but you can always learn and absorb something that is advantageous. No doubt, old theory is old theory. There are some out of date knowledge and information involved, but some of the good traditions have been experienced and tested by the generations of people, and some beneficial facts definitely can be produced to make desired achievement in life science. Traditional Chinese Medicine that has greatly loved and influenced the world, specially, the essential part as a preventive medicine like the Qi Gong exercises. The practitioner benefits from its produce and cultivate the body's energy to process the healing power of the body. This becomes a particular direction leading to health by many people in the world. The positive results and appreciation though Qi Gong, and Tai Ji Quan form exercise has gone far beyond any explanations that we can make in our current time. The only medical explanation could be - That Traditional Chinese Medicine theory affect a human's inner actions that awaken the power of the existent natural energy, Qi.

The natural makes the peace. The systems of the human body are not originally prepared to take so many kinds of processed productions such as strong medicines and supplements. The body's systems do not need to add so many newly invented "good things" of health products to keep it functioning. The body needs its own natural oils, nutrition, within its own network to stay supple, hydrated and healthy. The body's systems have their own natural ability to keep a good balance. If you add too many the unnecessary things, the body has to take its energy and time to fight-off the needless or useless additives that have entered it.

To be able to create balanced energy, each person should understand what their specific body's needs, and how to help these needs. However, everybody has special needs for their very own body, but one thing should be in common, that is, keeping and increasing the positive energy flow through all their organs to keep them functioning well everyday by staying active. We need to choose a way to exercise the body; and here, we will talk about how to choose certain kinds of motions and thoughts to support these organs system that work very hard for us. Favorably, many people have been practicing Qi Gong - a health promoting exercise that nurture and adjust our breathing, posture, and brings a greater focus.

Nurturing life is to exercise the body and power the mind to create a balanced energy. People getting sick shows that they are out of the balance. Most likely, is from not getting enough rest or relaxation for such a busy world, where everything goes faster and faster like the speed of a computer; the busy life unbalances the body and mind, courses an overly occupied mind and inactive body. Well, humans are not a computers and our energy is not generated electronically. We have our own pace to do things and to live, but some people forget, and their body is not sensitive enough to tell them to slow down and their emotions are tensely hurried with catching up with everything, everyday. This only ends with getting unhealthy.

We can always remind our self in this busy world that, "We cannot always direct the wind, but we can adjust the sails," which is to find our relaxed response to this stressful world. Each of our bodies has this ability and we just need to recognize and trust it. In this Chinese Medical Qi Gong practice, we will learn to use postures and movements through the knowledge of understanding the meridian channels to be able to cultivate more Qi, energy in the body, to prevent disease, to heal the illness, and to recover quicker and to have a healthier body.

Qi, also can energized the brain because the brain is part of the body. Energy is well balanced or imbalanced can be expressed in our feelings. For instance, why am I so depressed? Why am I so anxious? Why am I so fearful? These all show an imbalanced state of the mind that reflects our feelings. When you are depressed, may be because you live in the past and cannot let go of the negative things of the past. Sometimes, you may be anxious, because you fantasy the future without thinking realistically. You may be so fearful from time to time, because you may not ready for what you wished for, and simply need to be better prepared. These are symptoms of unbalanced Qi, negatives controlling the positives. Such unbalanced emotions effect the body physically. The longer time you hold on to these negative feelings, the more likely they could cause serious mental and physical diseases.

If we all can simply be more relaxed, our lives would improve and through the help of Qi Gong exercise, we will have a greater chance to create more relaxed thoughts, that lead to happiness, because you are less nerves, have less fear, and less worry, and are defiantly, sick less.

The Dao is near, but everybody looks far away. Staying healthy should be a lot simpler than getting sick, but many people take very complicated ways to take care of themselves, and forget the basics, which simply are three things for physical living: eating good, sleeping well, and exercising every day - these are good enough to keep the body's natural responsiveness, and adaptability in mental action. Health is like everything else, if there are no basics, there is no way to go further.

Preventive Medicine:

"It is too late to just start to dig a well when you feel thirsty." - A Chinese proverb.

"It is always better to understand your own illness rather than only relay on your doctors; focusing on daily health is better than paying attention to your health only after you are sick." - A Chinese proverb.

Prevention, is commonly not understood or included in medicine in most people's mind, because prevention is not a drug, surgical procedure or extensive lab test. People's mind and society are mostly focused on treating disease, and pay much less attention to prevent getting sick. The point is why not prevent instead of having to cure?

Traditional Chinese Medicine has been accepted commonly and practiced practically as one of the alternate treatments in the West, so does in China: there are considerable number of all kinds of the over-the-counter Chinese medicines are picked when people don't feel well – a quick way of curing. Of course, the alternative is a fantastic option to cure diseases, but the central core and meaning of Chinese Medicine should be more than expected, which is its Qi flow and power of prevention and healing. In the point of fact, preventive is respectfully recognized by whose long time practitioners and whoever really understands the most essential part of the Traditional Chinese Medicine - they practice the energy work to cultivate the Qi, nurture the spirit, and keep its flow and balance in daily life as a life style! In Chinese culture, we say: "The greatest ideal of Tradition Chinese Medicine is 治末病 Zhi Mo Bing, as its highest understanding and practice level." Zhi Mo Bing means, "the best method of medicine is that cures before the disease can enter the body,"

"The most effective medicine is preventing all the negative attacks to win a ill free life!

You may think if a medicine is not going to focus on the treatment of illness, it should not to be called medicine. You may be partly right, because Chinese Medicine is not like Western medical systems that look for the treatment as a goal. Since the Traditional Chinese Medicine was invented thousands of years ago, it might not have the solutions to all the modern diseases, during its long time development, the "medicine" is always focused on harmonizing the body, and balancing the body's energy. Even strong herbs that are used for serious conditions are still based on balancing the imbalances of the body's energy. Simply look at it this way: it is not the same thing as western medicine that could possibly save a life by surgical technologies and strong medicine treatments. Chinese medicine has its limitations, but so do all kinds of medicine, but Chinese medicine may be advanced in preventing disease through human's natural body abilities to correct its own disordered system functioning.

Through its thousands of years of developmental history, Traditional Chinese Medicine has focused on three parts, that I will go into and I'll also make a general comparison to Western medicine:

Part one: Preventive.

In Chinese medicine: Eating seasonal food to provide energy and nourishment is basic. Anything taken into the body is in accord with human's needs of growing physically and supporting thoughts. Food is a fundamental of healthy living, and ingesting proper foods is a daily process to prevent from disease and promote anti-aging.

Living in harmony with nature: Starting a day when the sun rises; resting begins when the sun sets - this follows the laws of nature as well as regulating the inner body's balance of the Yin and Yang.

A Chinese saying: "Activities enhances life," exercise the body and mind through Qi Gong, Tai Ji Quan, and martial arts to cultivate the body's energy and strengthen the internal organs and systems. "Prevention has always been considered more important and comes before treatments" as most Chinese folks known.

In western medicine: This part may be compared to the Western programs of exercise and diet. These programs don't belong to Western medicine, instead, it is to the general field, simply known as "Fitness."

Part two: the Earlier the treatment, the better the result.

In Chinese medicine: Balancing the body's Qi, and enriching the blood with the treatments of acupuncture, massage, cupping, and the usage of light herbs adjust the imbalances and restore positive Qi, energy to help the patient recover the from illness the soonest.

In Western medicine: Taking pills.

It makes logical sense that strong medicine is not good for a pure body, either Chinese medicine or western. When the Western medicine enters the body and stops the pain, it is a very useful tools in treating illness and changing the patient's health situation, proven by research and testing. When the Chinese medicine enters the body, the medicine's ingredients starts to work on the imbalance of energy to treat depressed organs and reduce symptoms. It may take much longer time to get the results than Western medicine, because Chinese medicine is trying to treat the root of the disease that the doctor found in the patient's body and regulate the irregularities. Both Chinese and Western medicine have side effects depending on the individual, and some times for some people, sadly, both medicine don't work as expected.

Part three: Take a chance.

In Chinese medicine: The strongest combinations of herbs are used for serious diseases.

In Western medicine: Currently, the greatest technologies that the whole world are developing and using to save lives when lives are really in danger.

The above show the strong points of Chinese medicine that is its preventive stage which depends more on a human being's lifestyle; while

Western medicine's strong point is its advanced technology. These three stages of medical practice respond to a person's health. The focus changes when the health conditions change. If we constantly put our priority on the first part and preventive medicine, our health will stay on top.

Qi, as a natural medicine is centered on living a healthy life style, that simply will enable us to sense and recognize whether our energy is in good balance or not, and lead us to the best natural "medicine" that protects us and nourishes us like using the most natural "herbs" to feed our own needs. That is why the Chinese saying "The prevention is more important than curing." Besides, healthy is a personal concern, an individual responsibility. There is also a Chinese proverb saying: "It is too late to just start to dig a well when you feel thirsty." That expresses effectively the truth of good health. As a practitioner who dedicate to seek the solution to health problems and gain a healthier life, this thought vividly in my mind all the time, in which, the full quality of practicing Chinese medicine is not only focused on the treatment as the only goal, but the value of useful preventive practices.

Unfortunately, many times in life, many people are losers in the battle for superior health. For instance, when you are sick, all your wish is to recover as quickly as you can, joining the fight against illness with common pills of Chinese or Western medicine, and waiting and trying to get "right one" that works, but some of them, unluckily, just don't work. There are come bodies don't have good respond all-time to all the medicines. Because one's complicated insides can be very different from others. Since medicines made from the same formulas are for solutions to a common problem, and often don't address specific personal problems. Meanwhile, pills still seem to be the best solution, easiest way to depend on at some points. So the body follows the procedure that the medicine indicates. Some people heal quickly, some do not. This is partly because the body has an individual nature with a formula of its own that has an inside pattern that responds to formalized medicine differently, getting different results from different medicine usage. This depends on how quickly your body's system can regulate your Qi, energy to its best level with the help of the medicine. If you can quickly build up the body's system closer to its regular and balanced energy level, the illness cannot destroy you completely. Positive energy will provide you the power to defeat the illness by taking the best from medicine and win the battle with disease fairly quick to regain good health again. The point here is: Qi is an inside helper.

Medical Qi Gong can be one of the most important components, in a health program, that acts like a powerful preventive medicine, because Qi Gong is not only based on the guiding and cultivating the energy through the meridian channels, but also includes some very special elements within its practice, such as the consciousness of the mind, the deep level of breathing, and the body alignments combined with the slow and steady rhythm of the movements. These combinations cultivate Qi through the body's meridian channels, that, in turn, lead practitioners a pleasant feelings as if watching a gentle water flow through a river. This is not the same feeling that walking or any other kind of workout exercise can provide. Qi Gong exercises stand on their own principles and apply them in motion, including a high quality stage of awareness in which we find connections between the body and mind, thereby changing practitioners from hardness and stiffness into a strong, yet soft and elastically flexible human being.

Especially, the medical Qi Gong, that helps us and protects us as natural medicine and is produced, not through laboratories and factories, but by our own natural energy, that we get from food, sleep, and exercise. The stronger the energy a person has, usually, the stronger immune system he or she will have, the less sick he or she will get. This is all because the meridian channels open up with Qi flowing through them, so the related organs get stronger support from the Qi Gong exercise. That explains why Qi Gong can heal and prevent illness. Many times, constant bad health is not because the diseases are not curable, but because people witness their own health only in a very late, complicated stage where no longer have many medical choices left.

One of the Chinese medicine greatest point views on health is that prevention is always a more important step for health than just finding a way to cure the illness. To be healthy is everybody's priority, it's been said in Chinese: "Focusing on daily health is better than only paying attention to your health when you are already sick," and, "it's better to understand your own illness rather than only relay on your doctors." In other words, repairing the body and organs obviously can never become the first choice for being healthy. That only downgrades one's quality of living, and gives no choice but living the best one can, with their health conditions. If you understand this simple way of thinking, you should act everyday for your health. We also have to understand that Qi Gong is a way of exercise. It may not be as the highly respected as medical procedures that can save people's lives, but it has a practical value of a way of operating, that at its least, politely opens the door to experience a healthier way of living, and help to win the battle in living a healthier, simpler life verses a complicated diseased life.

Of course, science is the guide of life and health. The goal of both Chinese and Western medical science is to achieve higher knowledge and more of it all the time. The processing of attaining greater knowledge and achievements will never end, and both medicines have good value in health field, as well as they both have their own theories to balance within their own specialized development. However, the Dao is always near you and life sciences are based on life itself. A human life should be more expensive than the price of doing medical procedures. Health should have more value than the cost of any materials. Everybody should be a responsible researcher into their own life and health, because you want to live your life better, not others! Therefore, Qi, plays as a great and sensitive messenger who deliver the truth of one's health from one's inside.

Chapter 2

A Short History of Traditional Chinese Medicine
- All the great theory we know now is from the past...

Traditional Chinese Medicine, also known as TCM, is a traditional medical practice originating in China. Although well-accepted in the mainstream of medical care throughout East Asia, it is getting popularly considered as an alternative medicine practice in the Western world, especially, acupuncture, which has the highest acceptance everywhere.

Like most of Chinese traditional cultures, Chinese medicine was mainly practiced within family lineage systems, that are all based on the same, or similar principles of ancient philosophy; theories of Yin-Yang, the Five-elements, the Zang-Fu, the meridian-channel-system, etc. Different traditional family systems had their own styles and specialties in treatments, especially on the usage of the herbs. This is because the diagnoses of the diseases were only made through the doctor's personal skill and experience, so each individual had to be treated differently.

The classical Chinese philosophy that forms Daoist thoughts also forms the philosophy of Chinese medicine, which reflects the classical Chinese belief in which the life and activity of an individual human being has an intimate relationship with the natural environment on all different levels. Since the first ever Chinese Medicine book, the "Yellow Emperor's Classic of Internal Medicine" was written in the 476-221 B.C. All kinds classical medical practices heavily rely on classical medical books and theories and methods dated from before the fall of the Qing Dynasty (1911). In Chinese history, this was also the peak time of the Chinese martial arts, especially the Internal Martial Arts are popularly practiced by many people to promote their health. Not until the 1950s, under the people's Republic of China, was Chinese medicine systematized to the public; including herbal medicine, acupuncture, Tui Na, Qi Gong and Tai Ji Quan practices are closely associated with TCM. Therefore, Chinese medicine and Qi Gong have a long relationship in history.

Now, let's go back to when it all stated.

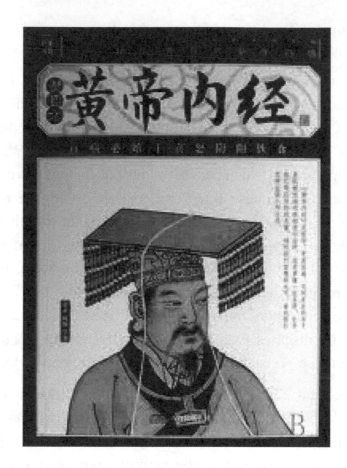

Figure 2-1

The first Chinese Medical book, the "Yellow Emperor's Classic of Internal Medicine" was written about 2500 years ago (Figure 2-1). It serves as a symbol of and a guide to the foundations of the traditional Chinese medical system. This first Chinese medical book is a reflection of medical science accomplishments in China during the Warring States Period (476-221 BC). It is not a product of any single person in any single period. This fantastic work explains the principles of the laws between the universe and life. Studying this book one not only to learn how to treat the patients, but also learn from this great mentor to understand the nature of wisdom that has profound knowledge to nurture all livings on Earth.

In this greatest of medical books in ancient China, meridian theory was established and defined as the core of a human being's health, it is described in there: "Meridians are the foundation of life, they also are the reason for causes of illness, as well as why the illness can be cured." The meridian system not only involves the Qi and blood channels, but also can balance Yin and Yang to protect and nourish the tissues and bones. The purpose of the use of acupuncture needles, herbs, or exercises, is stimulating and balancing the Yin and Yang energy through the meridians channels. Through this all illness could be cured. Through such strong belief and research, the TCM system has developed through generations as known as the medical classics.

The "Yellow Emperor's Classic of Internal Medicine" expounds many principles of harmony among humans and nature, physiology, anatomy, pathology, diagnosis, regimen, prevention, treatment of diseases, and so on, materialistically and dialectically. It has become the foot stones of Chinese medical science, the source of the theoretic system of traditional Chinese medicine, and the basis for clinical diagnosis of various diseases. Thus, later generations regard it as the "The most classical medical book," "The foundation of Chinese medicine." A necessary book for all the enthusiasts and students of Traditional Chinese Medicine.

They were many famous doctors in Chinese medical history. All of them had been working really hard and served the rich or poor, and all of their medical practices based on the ideas of the yellow emperor's medical classic, as well as having established their own styles through their own experiences, at their own times and contributed their own knowledge to the Traditional Chinese Medicine system.

Here are some famous doctors in the Chinese medicine history, of cause, they were many, many more who worked in the development of this tradition.

Hua Tuo

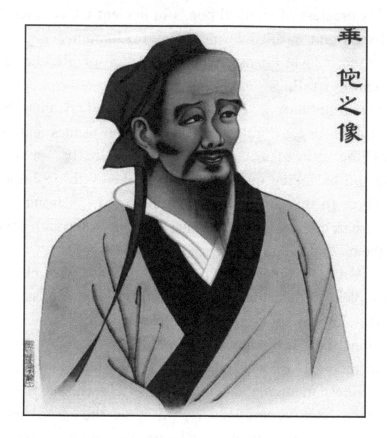

Hua Tuo

In the Han Dynasty, Hua Tuo 华佗 (110-207), was an outstanding medical Doctor, known as the "Father of Traditional Chinese Medicine." Hua Tuo had a habit of reading, studying different areas of knowledge in his youth. He was interested in knowing all kinds of classics and health sciences. When he grew a little older, he declined conscription into the court to work as an officer, and focused instead on keeping practicing medicine among the common people for a long time, and his footprints covered many places including present-day Anhui, Shandong, Jiangsu, Henan and other provinces in China. He was deeply respected and loved by the people.

Hua Tuo was not only skilled in acupuncture, obstetrics, gynecology and pediatrics, but also in internal medicine and other aspects of high attainments. His greatest success was in the surgical field. He is famous for making an herbal formulae, Ma Fei San, and successfully using it to keep a patient under general anesthesia in abdominal surgery. According to historical records, Hua Tuo was able to remove tumors, and perform a class of gastrointestinal surgical suturing. He used surgery on patients whose diseases could not be cured with acupuncture and medication. When using surgery, he let the patients served Ma Fei San wine, drink until they were unconscious. Then he opened their abdominal wall cut out the tumor and removed the dirty parts of the disease. Then after washing the wound the patient was good to be sutured and the wound dressed with a healing ointment. Forty-five days after the wound healed, the patient's health was restored. After that, Ma Fei San became a traditional medicine used as a general anesthetic. This all happened 1600 years before the use of general anesthetics in the West. Hua Tuo was way ahead of his time with his invention of a general anesthetic.

He also focused on physical exercise to help people's health. He had researched the physical activities of animals specifically the characteristics of the Tiger, Deer, Bear, Monkey and Bird. Then, He combined the theory of the energy flow and distribution of energy through the meridian pathways with the physiological functions and pathological changes of the human body, and the relationship between the movements of these five animals and the five major inner organs of the human body: the Heart, Liver, Kidneys, Lungs, and Spleen. Using this information from his research, he invented this set of exercises, which he proudly called: "My Doctor," or "the Dr. who takes care of my own health." The Five Animals Frolics, or Wu Qin Xi in Chinese, was first documented in a chapter of the "Three Kingdoms Period - Biography of Hua Tuo," by Chen Shou, during the Western Jin Dynasty (A.D.265-316). Hua Tuo was one of the first people, in the world, to use movements as a healing art.

The ancient health art of Five Animals Frolics Qi Gong has continued to be practiced and has benefited people's health for over 1800 years. Practitioners use this physical and mental exercise to increase their Qi accumulation, protect and strengthen their internal organ's functions and the prevention and cure of mental and physical diseases.

Zhang Zhong Jing

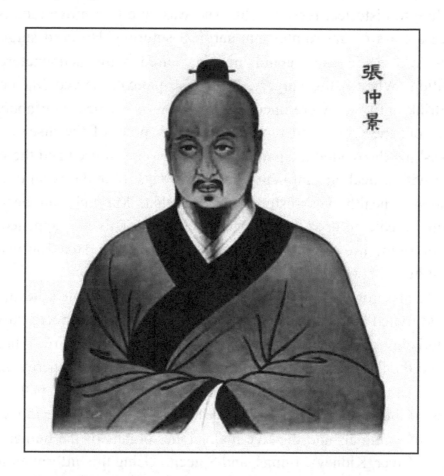

Zhang Zhong Jing

Zhang Zhong Jing was born in Nan Yang City, He Nan Province in the Eastern Han Dynasty (25-220 AD). It is said that he was once conferred an honorary title by the court and worked as the satrap of Changsha. Zhang Zhong Jing had been fond of medical science since childhood, and learned medicine from Zhang Bo Zu as they lived in the same county when he was young. After many years of hard learning and clinical practice, he won high prestige and became an outstanding medical scientist in China.

In the last years of the Eastern Han Dynasty, a prevalent pestilence claimed the lives of thousands. According to records, from the first year of the Jian An region (196), two-thirds of people died of infectious diseases in just one decade, of which febrile diseases caused by cold accounted for seventy precent.

Zhang Zhong Jing diligently learned from the book of the Yellow Emperor Internal Medicine, and collected prescriptions extensively. As a result, he wrote the monumental work, "Treatise on Febrile Diseases Caused by Cold and Miscellaneous Diseases." The principle of treatment according to symptoms differentiation established in this book is the basic rule of clinical medicine in China, and the soul of traditional Chinese medicine. In the study of prescriptions, the book "Treatise on Febrile Diseases Caused by Cold and Miscellaneous Diseases" has made a great contribution, too: it has created numerous types of recipes, and recorded many effective formulas. The principle of treatment according to the six channels, established in the book, has been highly regarded by doctors of all generations. It is the first monographic medicine work in China which established the principle of treatment according to symptoms differentiation from theory to practice. It is one of the most influential works in the history of Chinese medicine. Thus, it has become a fundamental textbook for medical study in later generations, and been highly valued by both medical students and clinical doctors.

There is a paragraph in the book that reads, "The medicine will be scrved as one purpose: that should be only used for curing nobles, save the poor, and keep everyone in good health." This shows the kindheartedness of Zhang Zhong Jing as a great doctor, as well as a clear definition of the meaning of the Traditional Chinese Medicine! So later generations grant him the honorific title: "Saint of Medicine."

Sun Si Miao

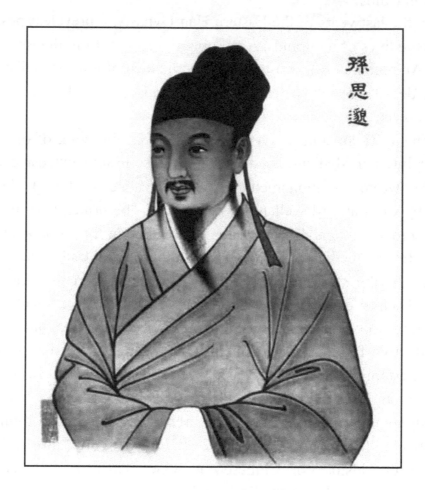

Sun Si Miao

Sun Si Miao (581-682) was a wonderful medical scientist in China in the Tang Dynasty (618-907). He was a native of Jiang Zhao, now Sun Jia Yuan in Hui County, Shan Xi Province.

Sun Si Miao's viewpoint on medical ethics was very important in the history of Chinese medicine. In his Qian Jin Yao Fang "Essential Prescriptions Worth a Thousand Pieces of Gold." He put forward the notion of "good faith of a great doctor" for the first time, offering an all-round argumentation on the guiding rules of medical ethics that a doctor must hold to. "Human life is of paramount importance, more precious than a thousand pieces of gold and to save it with one prescription is to show your great virtue." His book was named as "Qian Jin Yao Fang" (Essential Prescriptions Worth a Thousand Pieces of Gold), which was just a manifestation of such a noble moral character. He gathered and studied the medical data before the Tang Dynasty, and concerning his own clinical experience of several decades, he wrote Bei Ji Qian Jin Yao Fang "Essential Prescriptions Worth a Thousand Pieces of Gold for Emergencies," and Qian Jin Yi Fang "Additions to the Prescriptions Worth a Thousand Pieces of Gold," which have 30 volumes each.

Sun Si Miao paid great attention to women and children's care and wrote "The Prescriptions for Women" in three volumes and "The Prescriptions for Children and Infants" in two volumes, which were taken to be the beginning of the "Essential Prescriptions Worth a Thousand Pieces of Gold."

In pharmacology, he collected many empiric methods, used for processing, classifying and storing of drugs.

Sun Si Miao's study on health care was very profound. He advocated putting prevention of diseases at the first place, stressed the importance of "restraining desires to cultivate mental poise," "caution in speech," and "moderate in eating." All such ideas can serve as a good reference for the present-day gerontology.

One of the greatest accomplishments of Sun was the making of a set of chart with the 12 primary meridians and 650 acupuncture points. That was the first time in history, the doctors or people who were interested in medicine had an identified picture that showing the meridians and acupuncture points clearly. It indicated 48 single point and 301 double points with 349 names of the points. All together, there were 282 points in the front (Figure 2-2), 194 points in the back (Figure 2-3), and 174 points on the side (Figure 2-4).

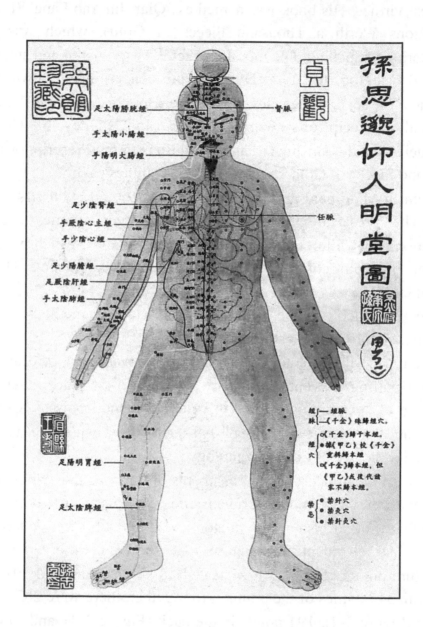

Figure 2-2

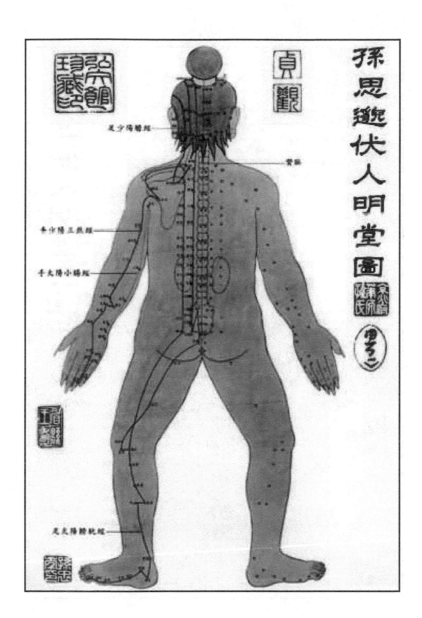

Figure 2-3

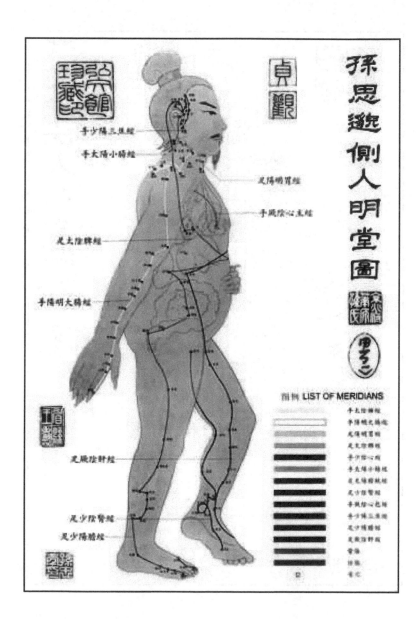

Figure 2-4

Li Shi Zhen

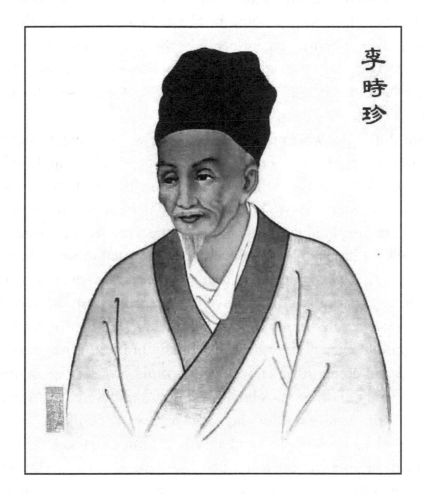

Li Shi Zhen

Though unknown in mainstream American culture, Li Shi Zhen (1518-1593), Ming Dynasty, is virtually a household name in China. A kind of patron saint of Chinese herbal medicine, widely lauded by historians and practitioners of Traditional Chinese Medicine., He is widely represented in popular and scholarly media nowadays as a very impressive sixteenth-century doctor who lived, worked, and died in south China.

Li was born in an area now known as Qi Chun in Hu Bei Province. His grandfather had been a traveling doctor, his father was a doctor, and that appeared to be his career path as well. He studied the medical classics, apprenticed with his father, treated local townsfolk, and eventually became successful enough to secure some brief yet high-profile positions in the capital and to befriend a few influential scholars. He wrote several short medical treatises on everything from mugwort to pulse diagnosis, composed some poetry, and made a decent living for himself, his wife, and his sons.

But this is not what put Li's face on the walls of medical colleges if he had not spent the last half of his life researching and writing an enormous book that became his magnum opus, the book "Ben Cao Gang Mu," an encyclopedic work in the traditional literature of herbs, which includes works explaining the qualities of the various substances used in making medical drugs: plants, animals, and assorted other materials. This book is one of the most ancient forms of medical writing in China that took Li decades of his life time, traveling, learning from farmers, hunters and local healers, and trying various treatments for his own patients until he had compiled enough information to satisfy himself. Then was the time to sit down and compose an encyclopedia of his own. He spent more than ten years writing his enormous book, and perished before it was published. Only due to the hard work, editing, and perseverance of his son and his disciple, was Li's book finally printed in 1596, three years after his death.

What an amazing book it was! The largest and complete work on medical material of his time, the "Ben Cao Gang Mu" contains 52 chapters of descriptions, stories, poems, histories, and recipes for how to use and understand everything from fire and mud to ginseng and artemisia, turtles and lions, and even human body parts as medical drugs. Li was a obsessed man who thought the only way to properly use something as a drug was to understand as much as possible about it. He stuffed everything he could find into his book, from as many different books as he could get his hands on.

Li's name and story have been resurrected many times since his death to serve many different purposes. In posters and films, he was recast in the image of a wandering people's doctor in the 1950s. As a result, most people today know of him as the father of Chinese pharmacology. Many TCM colleges in China, and scientists continue to test his recipes and translate his sixteenth-century pharmaceutical insights into the drugs and terminology of modern biomedicine.

Wang Wei Yi

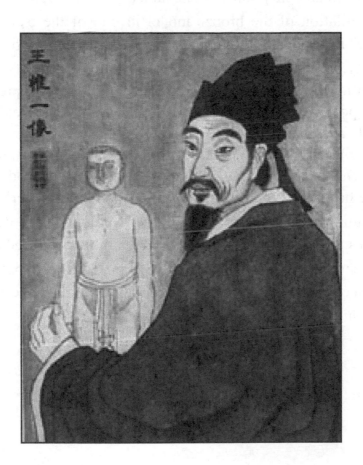

Wang Wei Yi

Wang Wei Yi was a famous physician in the Song Dynasty. Using his Illustrated Manual of the Practice of Acupuncture, and his support from the Government, Wang made two life-size bronze models with bronze details of the various points marked on the body. This helped in the standardization of acupuncture techniques. Explaining these points, Wang also wrote a book, and had the contents of the book carved on the surface of a few stones. After the wars of the Song Dynasty, the copper models and the surface of the stones were brought from the South to the North, but the bronze models and the stones later were found to be missing. Only some scattered pieces were left in the hands of some common people. One piece of the original collection of stone tablets is in the Beijing museum, as well as an imitation of the bronze model in one of the exhibition halls. This "bronze" is not made from copper, but uses gypsum in the style of the Ming Dynasty bronze system. (Figure 2-5).

The original bronze is 1.73cm high, and 345 holes representing the acupuncture points filled with mercury. If an acupuncture needle went into the point hole accurately, mercury would come out. There were organs and bones inside of the model that were caving vividly. Most important, the 12 meridian channels were very accurately laid out on the model's body.

There have been countless doctors, researchers, and common people who were natural resources and because they were interested devoted their time and lives to bring out the possibilities of a more advanced or effective state in ancient and modern China. There is no single person's work that would be successful without other's help. Chinese medicine is the same way and has involved generations of hard work.

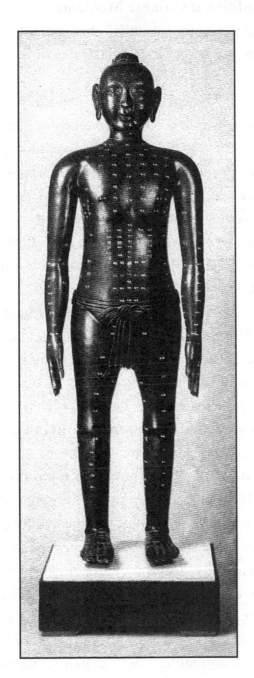

Figure 2-5

Understanding Traditional Chinese Medicine

Here, I'd like to briefly introduce this ancient art, to my the best of my ability, in a clear and readable format that will be easy for everyone to understand.

The Traditional Chinese Medicine, before western medicine was introduced into China, was the only medicine for the Chinese people for thousands of years. Even in today's China, along new research and development, TCM is an extremely rich discipline, built upon the combined experiences of famous practitioners of past dynasties, and the extensive books of medical writings they produced.

In Han Dynasty, a medical book of "Culture and Arts," defined Chinese Medicine as "The skills in Chinese medicine are to make people a quality, long, and healthy life."

Also, in late Han Dynasty, another famous medical doctor Guo Yu Zhuan talked about Chinese medicine as "医者，意也," "A good doctor, who must have to be mindful." It means, as a doctor who treats the human body, he must have a great philosophy and his own high spiritual and clear consciousness that qualifies him to help people in understanding nature and their own body's Qi, and to help people living a life correctly, attain superior health, and achieve longevity.

The theories of TCM at this point are quite different from those of Western medicine. TCM considers nature and human beings to be unified as a whole, and emphasizes the philosophical concept known as "The Unity of Heaven and Man." 天人合一. Environmental factors such as the four seasons, and changes in temperature and weather are believed to influence the human body, that the body and nature forming an integrated system. For instance, when the weather is suddenly hot in the spring, humid in the summer, dry in the fall, or cold in the winter, TCM employs treatments known as "eliminating fire," "expelling dampness," "moistening the body," and "guarding against cold" respectively. A simple way to understand this is: each one of us is a small Yin and Yang, and expected to harmonize with the big Yin and Yang of the universe.

Traditional Chinese Medicine also believes that every organ of the body has their own Qi. All organs and systems of the body are considered to be closely connected and mutually interacting. "The outside of the body is Yang, the inside is Yin; the back is Yang, the abdomen is Yin." TCM uses Yin-Yang Theory, Five-Elements Theory, and Organs-Theory, which advocate "administering treatment according to a pattern," rather than "treating the head when the head hurts; treating the foot when the foot hurts." According to the Five Elements Theory, the liver and gallbladder are Wood, the heart is Fire, the spleen and stomach are Earth, the lungs and intestines are Metal, and the kidneys and bladder are Water. When the Yin and Yang of the elements is out of balance, disease and disorder result.

Since Chinese medicine is deeply related to the whole body system, understanding the patient's attitude and outlook become a base of the tools that help the doctor's in diagnosis and treatment. Classical TCM believes that a person's visible surface, reflect one's insides. Accordingly, Chinese medicine doctors use various diagnostic methods to get full and detailed information about their patients to guide their treatment. The diagnosis relies on inspecting the patients through their complexion, 望, smelling their breath, 闻, inquiring about their symptoms, 问, and feeling their pulses, 切, in a very detailed manner to determine the overall condition of the patient's body. These are also known as the four major methods, each having a distinctive function. Doctors could make a correct analysis of diseases by applying all of them. This was a wisdom of ancient times, before the development of the chemical testing for identifying or detecting disease. The skills of Chinese medicine system of pulsing is a completely different from a checking the pulse in the Western medicine. In Western medicine, pulsing is a way of counting the beats of the heart. The pulse checking in TCM, is to feel the reaction of the activities in the meridians to understand the patient's inner health, and listen to the talking that a life can give without language!

Traditional Chinese remedies consist of natural preparations. Several thousand years of experimentation have determined the specific medicinal properties of numerous herbs, and the specific prescriptions and treatments that should be used for a wide range of conditions. Traditional Chinese remedies may either be taken internally or applied externally to promote the recovery of normal functioning, accordance to the theory of "administering treatment according to patterns."

According to the Traditional Chinese medicine view, a vital energy called Qi flows through the body along the meridian channels. The health and illness is modulated by the flow of the Qi, or stagnation of Qi. The treatment is to balance the Qi. For example, one has memory loss: To Traditional Chinese Medicine, this would be viewed as a bladder channel problem; because this major Yang energy meridian transfers Qi throughout the whole body as well as around the top of the head and down through the spine and leg to the little toe. So, a TCM doctor would consider that the Yang energy cannot reach to the top of the head, so the lack of the support of Yang Qi becomes the source of the diagnoses, and the treatment will be based on restoring the Yang Qi. It is very challenging to define Qi in Western terms and understand culturally what Qi is. Because the word runs deeply through not only Chinese medicine, but also through Chinese art, literature, philosophy, martial arts, and the entire culture of Chinese life.

The treatments of TCM include different works as the follows:

Acupuncture 针刺: using a very fine needle inserted into the body according to the points on the meridian channels.

Body message 推拿: as known as Tui Na, a body work focuses on releasing the tension of the body and helping the flow of positive energy in the meridians to balance imbalanced energy.

Cupping 拔罐: placing several glass (match-lit-heat) cups on the body as a heated pressure message.

Qi Gong 气功: an exercise to cultivate energy and heal the illness.

Herbs 方剂: herb medicine used for treatment.

Therefore, the treatments above are still widely been practiced in China, but not used to retreat all kind of disease, commonly, good medical providers will give or suggest whatever the best for the patients, either Chinese or Western medicines. This is because the traditional methods that were invented and slowly developed in ancient times, absolutely have their limitations. To apply the entire method of the old TCM system to the treatment of all modern diseases is not a wise way to do things. It will make more sense that we take the Chinese system's very valuable preventive aspect to help people stay healthy. However, new diseases are continuously discovered and so are new medicines and new treatments continuously made and used both in Chinese and in Western medicines.

It's great to see more people have become interested in alternative lifestyles in recent years and there has been a corresponding upsurge of interest in Chinese medicine, herbal medicine and non-pharmaceutical treatments. Especially acupuncture and Qi Gong for health have become increasingly popular around the world. In the long run, the best medicine is still no medicine.

Understanding the Meridians in Chinese Medicine
Through its long history and complicated medicinal work, meridian theory has remained the central core of all the aspects and treatment methods of the Traditional Chinese Medicine.

• **The Creating of the Meridians** 经络
An ancient Chinese saying: "If meridian theory had not been invented, there would be no Chinese medicine, ever."

The meridians have a relationship with the organs, they reflect the functionality of the organs and their liabilities.

Everything comes out of nothing, the ancient Chinese call nothing, or emptiness *"Wu Ji."* It is nothing only because it has not developed yet, also as a concept of the potential for everything. Tai Ji is born from Wu Ji, making everything have their own opposite side, their own Yin and Yang; to accompany each other and make a whole object. This topic composes the central meaning of Chinese medicine. Yin and Yang are divided into four layers. They are greater Yin and greater Yang, and lesser Yin and lesser Yang. The early medicine book of "Su Wen" 素问, a part of the "Yellow Emperor's Internal Medicine" added absolute Yin and brightness Yang. So, each Yin and each Yang has three different layers. This was also based on the harmony of the treasures of the universe, heaven, earth, and man.

Thankfully, the ancient Chinese's imaginary abilities and creativity invented the meridian channels of the hand and foot. Each has three layers of Yin and Yang, totaling twelve meridians that circulate the body's energy and connect with the nature of the Heaven and Earth.

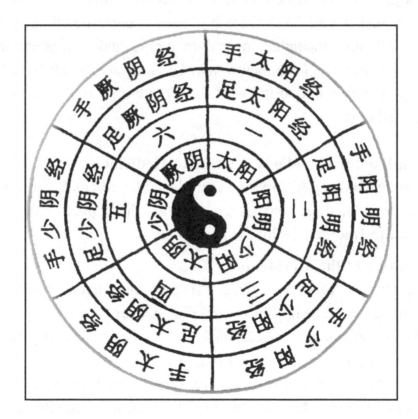

The body, as Chinese believed, employs the meridians to energize and repair the body and help it grow and develop and absorb nutrition from the food and movements of the activities in daily life Qi is the explanation of the process that creates and continuous polarizes the body's energy there by keeping the balance of Yin and Yang.

Here is a chart of the twelve primary meridians with their names, how they relate to Yin and Yang, and their correlations to hands and feet, as well their associations with the organs:

Meridian Name (Chinese)	Yin / Yang	Hand / Foot	Organ
Lung Meridian (LU) (手太阴肺经)	Greater Yin (太阴)	Hand (手)	Lung (肺)
Heart Meridian (HT) (手少阴心经)	Lesser Yin (少阴)	Hand (手)	Heart (心)
Pericardium Meridian (PC) (手厥阴心包经)	Absolute Yin (厥阴)	Hand (手)	Pericardium (心包)
Triple Burner Meridian (TB) (手少阳三焦经)	Lesser Yang (少阳)	Hand (手)	Triple Heater (三焦)
Small Intestine Meridian (SI) (手太阳小肠经)	Greater Yang (太阳)	Hand (手)	Small Intestine (小肠)
Large Intestine Meridian (LI) (手阳明大肠经)	Yang Brightness (阳明)	Hand (手)	Large Intestine (大肠)
Spleen Meridian (SP) (足太阴脾经)	Greater Yin (太阴)	Foot (足)	Spleen (脾)
Kidney Meridian (KI) (足少阴肾经)	Lesser Yin (少阴)	Foot (足)	Kidney (肾)
Liver Meridian (LV) (足厥阴肝经)	Absolute Yin (厥阴)	Foot (足)	Liver (肝)
Gallbladder Meridian (GB) (足少阳胆经)	Lesser Yang (少阳)	Foot (足)	Gall Bladder (胆)
Bladder Meridian (BL) (足太阳膀胱经)	Greater Yang (太阳)	Foot (足)	Urinary bladder (膀胱)
Stomach Meridian (ST) (足阳明胃经)	Yang Brightness (阳明)	Foot (足)	Stomach (胃)

- **What is Qi?**

Qi, has different meanings if used in short phases in Chinese language. Here, we are not going to research all the related meanings of Qi, rather it will be more efficient to move straight forward to an understanding of the meaning of Qi within our topics of Qi Gong and Chinese medicine.

Qi, here, means bodily energy related to a human's primary natural energy, or a cultivated, highly made energy. There are positive and negative energies. Qi is an activity or liveliness inside of the body that helps operates the function of bodily systems through the inner motion. A person's Qi can come into view and be visible for others to sense and see through his or her physical appearance or attitude.

Positive Qi is also a connection between the universe and human love, that can improve one's thoughts on many things in life. Negative Qi can destroy the harmony of the heart and spirit.

- **What Qi does in Medical Qi Gong?**

Qi Gong, is a combination of the breath, motion, focused mind exercises to cultivate a person's natural energy to its maxim potential to achieve a longer, healthier life. No matter what kind of Qi gong people practice, they are all related to Chinese culture, philosophy, martial arts and traditional medicine. All these practices are for the same purpose of getting stronger Qi in the body and spirit - the most important value that is involved in and influences all these arts.

Chinese Traditional Medicine is a culture and its theory is not easy to be understood well if you are not understood Chinese culture. Through the focus on studying the meridian theory, it'll help deepens the level of understanding and towards a better Qi Gong practice.

A directly conceived conception developed by the mind in ancient Chinese medicine is the theory of meridian channels. Medical Qi Gong practice is focused on the flow of Qi, energy throughout the meridian channels; thee channels are the energy pathways. The meridians are not like the organs that physically can be seen, but are perceived as a network of our energy in which we can feel, this is so called the Qi. Qi acts as an agent who provide with motivated gentle force to help transporting the blood and oxygen throughout the body, to enhance the function of the organs and stabilize one's health. Qi Gong practice is one who works on the Qi flow through a special exercise including the physical postures, movements, and mindset. Through continued processing, one must be to be able to feel their Qi, and direct it. The development of a higher level of Qi, will be taken so much time to practice to be successful.

First of all, the theory of the meridians must be understood as the connective support to all the organs, joints, bones, and external organs such as eyes, nose, mouth, and skin of the body, How to balance the Qi flow through the meridians that nourish the entire body system and adjust to the physical ability that comes with age, an individuals natural, and current conditions. To be able to make these kind of connections in the body, one will learn specific ways to move, to breath, and to be soft. These part need to be practiced diligently to gain progress and understanding; at the same time, practitioners must learn the fourteen meridian channels. Then, they will start to understand better their own Qi, and can apply these principles into their other practices.

The major function of Qi in medical Qi Gong practice, is to get stronger Qi in a balanced way. As a result of better Qi circulation and strengthens one's inner health to eliminate illness throughout human life, and serves as natural "medicine" that regulates the imbalances of the body and mind, and transforming them into healthier states. As a Chinese proverb says: "When the Qi is wrong, all the applications of medicament are of no use; when the Qi is correct, all chemical medicines are of no need."

Chapter 3

Qi Gong and Medical Qi Gong
Qi Gong

Qi Gong is a modern general term for energy work in China. Literally this translates into English as energy (Qi) work, and regularly practice to gain a special skill (Gong). In Chinese history, the development of modern Qi Gong has been associated with different schools or religions with their own related practice of breathing, meditation, guiding energy, as well the influence of their ideologies. Such as Chan 禅, in Buddhism; Ren 仁, in Confucianism; Jing Zuo 静坐, in Daoism; and Nei Gong 内功, in Chinese internal and external martial arts.

There are majorly four sets of Qi Gong that represent the major classical schools and are popularly practiced by people in China: They are the Five Animal Frolics, 五禽戏, The Six Healing Sounds, 六字诀, Da Mo's Muscle Change Classic 易筋经 and The Eight Brocades 八段锦. All these practices have one thing in common, that is, "Inner cultivation" based on a similar philosophy, but, also, all the religious groups and believers in the various philosophical systems have kept their own specific methods, terms, and versions of their practices, they continue to practice their own classical ways. However, based on historical documents, it is very clear that the thousands of years of practice in these disciplines strongly reflect the current understanding of Qi Gong.

For the time being, the influence of these practices from different groups of people have become widely accepted by more people in China. The term of "Qi Gong" formally and commonly started to be used as the art began to be practiced more in China was in the 1950s, along with Tai Ji Quan practice for health. Since then, people practice different Qi Gong forms and search for more Qi Gong forms from different areas where traditional Qi Gong is practiced by common folks. The true believers of Qi Gong for health have recently caught much attention for Qi Gong for the first time in the history, and more expected the art's helpfulness in the modern health care system. Thanks to these dedicated practices group and the continuous development of the art, this wonderful mind, body, and spiritual practice widely has increasingly accepted by people from different culture's backgrounds.

Medical Qi Gong:

There is no doubt that different kinds of Qi Gong practice can be very helpful for keeping practitioners healthy. Medical Qi Gong is even more credited as a healing art, which not only for being used as a modern term, but for its relationship to traditional Chinese medicine theory. Looking at the deep inner and essential connections between TCM and medical Qi Gong, we will see the aim of these two are similar, both are based on the ancient Yin and Yang philosophy, both are based on meridian theory, both share some methods of treatment, and both want to achieve the goal of being a preventive medicine. The medical Qi Gong that we are doing here, is a branch of Traditional Chinese Medicine; also greatly stands alone as a health preservation exercise that act directly to increase the natural healing power of the human body. Medical Qi Gong shares only some of the core fundamentals of TCM. As an art that cultivates the body's natural energy as "medicine," Medical Qi gong is not a replacement for the TCM system, rather confirms the logical principles shared by these culture arts.

Noteworthy is that Chinese Traditional Medicine is not always practiced like western medicine to treat patients when they have the problems. The high level of Chinese medicine is its "Prevention before disease happens." Its initial focus is not on how to treat illness with advanced medicine, instead of balancing energy to stay healthy. Simply, if you don't keep yourself healthy, you are not happy, you are limited in helping others.

Medical Qi Gong is a branch of Chinese medicine along with herbs, acupuncture, and Tui Na. Medical Qi Gong properly serves as a preventive medicine through Qi cultivation and balance. Clinically helps with recovery after the treatments by either eastern or western medical systems. Best of all, medical Qi Gong is not confined to a focus on treatments or recovery, it can be practiced alone as part of an exercise routine for your life, and, you are the boss to manage you time and your needs.

Since the Traditional Chinese Medicine doctor were not necessarily Qi Gong practitioners, Qi Gong or martial arts practitioners may not fully knowledgeable on Chinese medicine. A bridge of knowledge between these two great treasures should be built. Before we start to look at The Three Treasures medical Qi Gong, we need to understand a little more of how medical Qi Gong practices balance energy through the meridian theory of Chinese medicine.

Medical Qi Gong Manifest the Meridian Theory of TCM

The energy, or Qi, is not at the same level all the time in the body, it changes. Increasing and decreasing of the Qi level depends on the food eaten, sleep quality and activities of each day, it's very different within each individual. Qi Gong practice is a way of knowing yourself and naturally balancing the energy in the body. For example, when a person is sick because of a kidney Qi deficiency, she or he should practice some Qi Gong posture or routine that is good for cultivating Qi in the kidneys, rather than just practicing Qi gong breathing exercises over and over. Of course, the body's meridian network reaches everywhere of the body, one of the advantages of medical Qi Gong is its special motions that will focus and help certain areas of the body. Relatively speaking, this is somewhat similar to acupuncture treatments. For instance, when you take one session of acupuncture treatment that focuses on certain meridians with chosen points to stimulate or balance the energy in these meridians at that moment; a different focus of the treatment will be used in other sessions according to the conditions of the body's energy balance at that specific time. The difference between the treatment and Qi Gong practice is: acupuncture or massage are someone helping you, but Qi Gong is you helping yourself - an independent type of health care, which the increased sensitivity gained through your practice gives you a greater understanding about your own body, your own mind, and where these discomforts come from - these will give you right signals that will guide you do what you need to do. However, keeping yourself healthy is not really supposed to totally rely on doctors or professionals who give you treatments when you are not well, that could be little too late, it really should be about keeping a good balance of your own energy by yourselves for a true healthy life.

Medical Qi Gong in Clinical Application

A saying of the Yellow Emperor: "医者意也," Medicine is an extraordinary intensity of Doctor's mind."

The power of TCM lies within its meridian theory. Acupuncture uses the points to help to balance the energy along the meridians; message or Tui Na therapy works on certain areas of the body according to the meridians; Qi Gong practitioners cultivate their energy through the meridians; Qi Gong treatments designed for medical treatment also depend on the view of the functions of patient's meridians.

Medical Qi Gong practiced as a treatment is similar to clinical acupuncture and massage. Qi Gong therapists have to practice Qi Gong or Tai Ji Quan or related arts to high level to gain the special ability that much needed to give treatments to the patients. Because Qi Gong and TCM are not only limited to academic knowledge, but are about feeling the patient's energy, which can be felt through observation and pulsing made possible by the therapist's own energy and sensitivity. The higher the level of sensitivity, the more well balanced energy the therapist has, the better their energy connect to the patients. This leads to a more accurate process with more correct decisions on the treatments. However, to be a good Qi Gong clinician, the meridian study is rather than necessary as fundamental medical theory; regular Qi Gong practice is an essential. Although the skill is different from the skills of an acupuncturist or message therapist, additionally, these skills totally depend on the Qi Gong therapist's own ability to transport Qi to their patients.

Many people incorrectly believe that someone by putting their hands on their patient's body can start increase or complete the body's healing process. Unfortunately healing can never be as simply as that! In medical Qi Gong clinics, the ChineseTraditional Medicine knowledge of diagnosis and the ability to determine treatments according to the patient's individual differences has been, still is considered to be the basic training for qualified practitioners. Also as important as academic knowledge, is the medical Qi Gong therapist's own ability to prescribe Qi Gong exercises or a routine to the patients according the patient's specific medical needs. This part of clinical applications definitely has to be developed by the practitioner's own a long time energy practice, the clinical experience that have truly absorbed principles. Therefore, Qi Gong healing is a real creative process, that connects a person's energy flows as the therapist accurately applies Qi into the patients energy channels. This may be stronger, last longer than the treatment by acupuncture needles, because it comes with a human energy transmission.

In The Yellow Emperor's Classic it pointed out the significant concept that TCM practitioners should not be just a dispenser of herbs or just a treatment giver, "Yi Zhe Yi Ye 医者意也," this means, the practitioner should have gained a high level of intuition and ability of will, that makes them become those who see what the regular people do not see, feel what the average cannot feel, and transfer healing power that untrained people cannot transfer. This is first requires the clinician to have managed the TCM principles, that guide applications. For these principles to have become an unconsciousness reaction in treating their patients because the Qi must be in a well balanced stage in the clinician's physical body and mind, that harmonized with their heart and hands. Simply, if a person cannot see their own inner self, how can they sense and judge others correctly? This is a special qualification for being a higher level practitioner who feels the patients Qi as well as the problems, then, uses their own Qi to heal others. They are not limited by cold acupuncture needles inserted the patient's body, or some fixed formula herbs to feed their patients. The TCM or Qi Gong clinician must focus their own balanced Qi development all the time to gain the unique abilities of positive intension. Being physically healthy themselves is to give responsible help to their patients with a true Qi.

The World Earliest Qi Gong

The early Han period (early 2nd century BC) tombs of a noble family, excavated from 1972 to 1974 at Ma Wang Dui, Chang Sha, Hu Nan Province, China, are among the most important archaeological discoveries of the past quarter-century.

The tombs contained the remains of the Marquis Dai, his wife and son, and their most prized possessions. Over 3000 cultural relics and a well-preserved female corpse were unearthed, attracting wide attention home and abroad.

Among the relics were bright-colored lacquer wares representing the highest level of craftsmanship, fine silks showing amazingly accomplished weaving techniques, and inscriptions on silk demonstrating knowledge and wisdom of the ancient sages. Of all the remains, the most astonishing was the corpse of Xin Zhui, the spouse of the first Marquis of Dai, which was extremely well preserved. Most of the artifacts including the corpses can now be found in the Hunan Provincial Museum.

This is an exciting piece of silk with pictures illustrating in100cm wide and 40cm high, total of 44 "Dao Yin" postures that were found in tomb No.3. This is wonderfully proves that there were early Qi exercises for the healing effects of the movements. The Chinese characters located next to some of the posture figures explain the healing purposes of the postures and movements as the picture below:

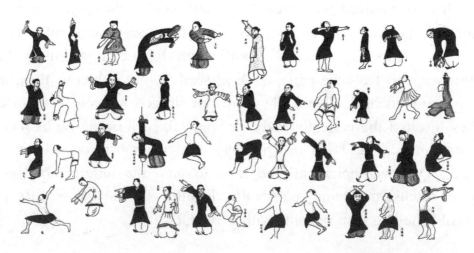

Chapter 4

The Three Treasures Qi Gong Form

Everybody deserves a gift to themselves, that will be a new understanding of your body, trusting your energy, and expanding the meaning of life.

Qi Gong's signature representation is the form practice. From ancient times to the present, there have been so many Qi Gong forms that it's impossible and unnecessary to learn all of them. Here are the reasons to learn this set of Qi Gong:

The Three Treasures Medical Qi Gong set establishes its own features within traditional Chinese medicine.

The Three Treasures Medical Qi Gong set has been thoughtfully formed of nine Qi Gong movements that are simple for everyone to learn.

The Three Treasures Medical Qi Gong set practice will efficiently cultivate one's inner energy and promote one's natural healing potential.

The Three Treasures Medical Qi Gong set is designed to teach the Chinese meridians in a practical way though a new learning processing.

The Three Treasures Medical Qi Gong set study is a wonderful learning experience of Daoist philosophy.

Before we start to learn the form, I would like to have a short note to explore the meaning of the acupuncture points names along the meridians, because the names of the points are not merely nominal, each has a profound meanings.

Traditional Chinese Medicine is a culture that is based on Daoism, and the careful observation of the geophysical connections of Heaven, Earth and Men have helped in the development of its own very special medical language. We first get to know there are 365 acupuncture points on the 14 meridians, each of the points has their meaningful name. They all appear commonly with their own two characters phase, a few have three characters when it necessary. Some of the names correlate with the phenomena of nature, some are described clearly by their locations on the body; some of them are classical information about the points; but one thing is in common, they all serve as a guides to help to memorize the points. For clinical treatments, there is much value in the names of the points. Some of the point names are telling reflect the situation of the inside of the body there, and some of them provide direct functional information as to the needles and pressures that should be used on the patients in treatments. Some of the point names fall into the category of information on energy in that area of the body, and all useful references in maintaining health.

Here are examples on how the Chinese characters are used to describe and relate to the point and its home channel.

KI1. Gushing Spring, 涌泉. The location is in the depression on the heart of the sole of the foot.

Explanation for this point: The sole of the foot is the lowest part of the human body, and the physical area connected to the Earth, where the spring water gushes from. For a deeper explanation of this point, is at the beginning of the water (kidney) channel, that gives life and Qi. All the sections of these Qi Gong postures and movements are based on focusing the stimulation of this important point to make connection to and absorb energy from the Earth.

GB21. Shoulder Well, 肩井。 The location is in the depression on the shoulder in front of the great bone.

Explanation for this point: The Yin and Yang culture shows the source of life and Qi coming from the Earth, which related the KI-1, Gushing Spring on the bottom of the foot; the water based human energy is always traveling upward and reaching the highest area of the shoulder, like a well that full of water. This also explains if the energy blockage happening any part of the body, the "well" cannot provide enough water to support the needs of life, the illness will occur.

Through the study these point names in Chinese and learning the meanings of the points will enable the practitioners understand the culture and history, easier to know how the body and mind connected, how to increase the energy flow inside of the body's systems, and how to use the points to stimulate the energy to treat the disease. The number classifications of the point names are a common way of studying the points for people who do not know Chinese language. They are the system that is used in this book; it shows the numbers right after the meridian abbreviations.

Obviously, there is neither a simple way to interpret all the meanings of the points in Chinese, nor is this the focus of the Three Treasures Qi Gong study. Since the more we know about the acupuncture points, the better we develop the relationship between academic knowledge and the feelings of our living bodies, we will learn on the meridian map through each sections of the Three Treasures Qi Gong practice. The Chinese character of the point will be written next to the acupuncture point's numbers for further study on their direct meanings as well as a source of reference.

In studying of this Qi Gong set, we concentrate on the knowing of the meridian channels rather than the acupuncture points. Because this Qi Gong practice is to intent for strengthening the meridian channels by the soft, expanded motions internally and externally, that serve the purpose of stimulating and helping energy flow throughout entire body. However, to achieve this goal, we need to know the starting and the ending points of each meridian to use the movements designed to open, lengthen, and unclog the meridians, only in this way, the Qi in the body can move and flow without obstruction. For people who are not interested in meridian study, there will be no difference in benefits of this Qi Gong practice. Without a study of the meridians, keep in mind, keep the principles well within your practice.

How to Follow This book for Self-study the Qi Gong Form:

Qi Gong cannot be done by understanding it intellectually, you need to practice until your body can appreciate your own energy. It may takes longer time than you think, but the learning and practicing only bring you a greater result, and you only get better!

The leaning processing from this book is in a format of three steps to learn and understand each section.

First, is the meridian study: it indicates the meridians that are involved in the section, some times more than one meridians need to be studied, or get familiar with.

Second, is to know the health benefits of the Qi Gong. This is focus on great benefits through strengthening the meridians that improve the functions of related internal organs. In this part, the meridian charts and name of the acupuncture points are listed in both in the code (like ST 36), and Pin Yin, and Chinese characters.

The third, is following by the explanation of the "Qi and Meridians" with image of the meridians which are the collection from the Ming Dynasty.

The fourth, is the explanations of the Qi Gong movement along the photos of each postures, step by step, by Tina Zhang.

The Three Treasures Medical Qi Gong Form

Heaven 天
1. Heaven Energy 乾气 (The Sun 日) 呼吸
2. Connecting to the Universe 自然 (The Moon 月)
3. Opening the Heart 畅心 (The Stars 星)

Earth 地
1. Balancing the Energy 舒中 (Water 水)
2. Strengthening the Essentials 强体 (Fire 火)
3. Flowing Earth Energy 坤气 (Wind 风)

Human 人
1. Cultivating Energy 补气 (Essence 精)
2. Harmony of the Three Treasures 和谐 (Qi 气)
3. Nurturing the Spirit 养神 (Spirit 神)

Heaven

"**Heaven gives the Yang energy to the human body that dominates one's health. Nurturing our life is nurturing our Yang Qi, that nurtures the soul and heart.**" - Tina Chunna Zhang

1. Heaven Energy 乾气

Meridian study:

Bladder, BL, 足太阳膀胱经, the longest meridian of the meridian channel system that contains 67points.

Health benefit:

Open the body's longest energy channel, breathing exercise, cultivate Yang energy, which is what mostly nurtures life.

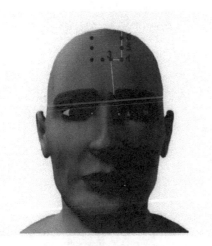 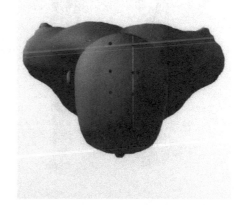

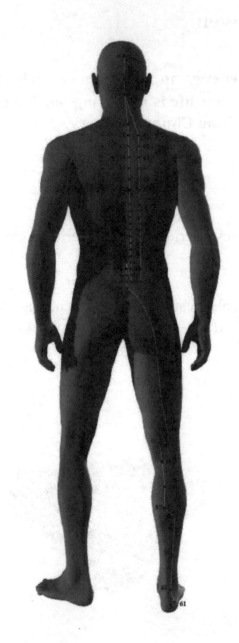

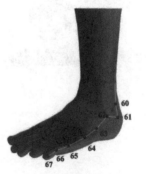

The Bladder Meridian, BL, originates from the inner side of the eyes, and passes through the forehead, flows down the back of the head, then, there it separates into two channels. One comes down about 3 Cun (inch) beside the mid-line of the center spine, down to the gluteal area. Another one runs straight downward to the lumber spine region, and continues along the leg down past the back of the knee, BL40, ending at the outside tip of the little toe. There are 67 acupuncture points of this meridian.

BL - Bladder Meridian 足太阳膀胱经

BL1 • Jing Ming 睛明

BL2 • Zan Zhu 攒竹

BL3 • Mei Chong 眉冲

BL4 • Qu Chai 曲差

BL5 • Wu Chu 五处

BL6 • Cheng Guang 承光

BL7 • Tong Tian 通天

BL8 • Luo Que 络却

BL9 • Yu Zhen 玉枕

BL10 • Tian Zhu 天柱

BL11 • Da Zhu 大杼

BL12 • Feng Men 风门

BL13 • Fei Shu 肺俞

BL14 • Jue Yin Shu 厥阴俞

BL15 • Xin Shu 心俞

BL16 • Du Shu 督俞

BL17 • Ge Shu 膈俞

BL18 • Gan Shu 肝俞

BL19 • Dan Shu 胆俞

BL20 • Pi Shu 脾俞

BL21 • Wei Shu 胃俞

BL22 • San Jiao Shu 三焦俞

BL23 • Shen Shu 肾俞

BL24 • Qi Hai Shu 气海俞

BL25 • Da Chang Shu 大肠俞

BL26 • Guan Yuan Shu 关元俞

BL27 • Xiao Chang Shu 小肠俞

BL28 • Pang Guang Shu 膀胱俞

BL29 • Zhong Lu Shu 中膂俞

BL30 • Bai Huan Shu 白环俞

BL31 • Shang Liao 上廖

BL32 • Ci Liao 次廖

BL33 • Zhong Liao 中廖

BL34 • Xia Liao 下廖

BL35 • Hui Yang 会阳

BL36 • Cheng Fu 承扶

BL37 • Yin Men 殷门

BL38 • Fu Xi 浮郄

BL39 • Wei Yang 委阳

BL40 • Wei Zhong 委中

BL41 • Fu Fen 附分

BL42 • Po Hu 魂户

BL43 • Gao Huan Shu 膏盲俞

BL44 • Shen Tang 神堂

BL45 • Yi Xi 意禧

BL46 • Ge Guan 隔关

BL47 • Hun Men 魂门

BL48 • Yang Gang 阳刚

BL49 • Yi She 意舍

BL50 • Wei Cang 胃仓

BL51 • Huang Men 盲门

BL52 • Zhi Shi 志室

BL53 • Bao Huang 胞盲

BL54 • Zhi Bian 秩边

BL55 • Hey Yng 合阳

BL56 • Cheng Jin 承筋

BL57 • Cheng Shan 承山

BL58 • Fei Yang 飞扬

BL59 • Fu Yang 跗阳

BL60 • Kun Lun 昆仑

BL61 • Pu Can 仆参

BL62 • Shen Mai 申脉

BL63 • Jin Men 金门

BL64 • Jing Gu 京骨

BL65 • Shu Gu 束骨

BL66 • Tong Gu 足通骨

BL67 • Zhi Yin 至阴

Qi and Meridian Channels

黄帝内经 告诉我们:天以气养人的阳.

    The Yellow Emperor's Classic tells us: "Heaven gives its Qi for human's Yang energy."

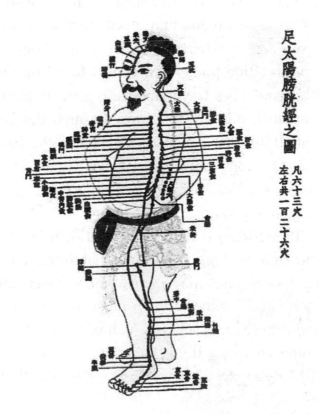

BL

According to Traditional Chinese Medicine, the **Bladder Meridian** has the most Yang energy of all the meridians. The Bladder Meridian runs from the head to the toes. Many points along this meridian are located next to the spine in the human body and they dominate the conditions of one's health. This is the longest meridian and strongest Yang channel in the body.

This meridian channel runs from the inner side of the eyes and flows up to the top of the head, BL7, a major acupouncture point, where the most Yang energy is gathered in this area. Straight up, naturally connects to the heavens, and is also the area of the brain. This meridians stores our Yang energy that we receive from the Heaven to nurture our life. However, nurturing our life is also, nurturing our Yang Qi.

The spine is composed of vertebras, that support our basic standing, sitting, and bending postures that we use every day in life. If you have certain curved areas in the back, or pain, it means that you have blocked Qi, or energy, in part of your BL meridian, which is also, sometimes, a symptom indicating some organs may need your attention due to their current lack of wellness. Therfore, many acupuncture points on this meridians are transportation points that conect to all the internal organs. Exercising the BL channel is a way to maintain general internal health.

The BL meridian also travels down through the back of the leg throught the point BL40, that helps relieve pain in the back through the practice of certain Qi Gong movements. The BL meridian ends at the outside of the tip of the little toe, which is the point, BL67, that helps women's monthly period and other fertility issues.

Since the BL meridian is the longest meridian in the body, it plays important role through its long connectng that bring the organs health together. Through Qi Gong movements and proper alignments, the practitioners would keep some of the most important energy points connected and make these areas active, which mobilizes the entire channel. Noticing these points and areas if you desire to, such as: BL7通天, BL9玉枕, BL11大杼, BL17隔俞, BL23肾俞, BL54 委中 (akaBL40), BL57承山, BL60昆仑, BL67至阴.

Working on the energy in our body should have an initial awareness of this meridian that conncts from the inner eyes to the little toes, in order to learn the strenghning of the entire Yang meridian that is formed by a natural connection, deeply related to the brain and central nervious system which runs along the spine that dominates a person's general health.

This meridian channel is not easy to open up by one's self sometimes; so a good massage along one's back is often neccessery to open up this spesific energy channel.

In this opening section of the Three Treasures Qi Gong, we are building smooth, and safe ladders that lead us all the way to the heaven, cultivating our natural energy and strenghning the Yang energy In our bodies.

Qi Gong Movement:
1. Heaven Energy (Heaven: 1 of 3)

Startig with a standing posture in an natural position (Figure 4-1). The body weight is on the right foot and left foot steps to the left side, about your shoulder's width or your hip's width (Figure 4-2). Starting place the hands/arms behind you on the level of lower back naturally, and the fingers of both hands are facing each other, and your hands probably are naturally in the area of BL28. Then coming up with palms facing forward with inhale (Figure 4-3, 4-4, 4-5). Place the bent elbows and hands behind the neck and upper back (Figure 4-6), where the BL meridian separates into two channels down the back and lower body, while exhaling. Your Arms continue to move upward reaching as high as you can, this strengthenes the upper back from BL13, up to the top of the head BL7, and is done while inhaling. Meanwhile, the body continues lengthening and focus stays on the back (Figure 4-7). Then, lift your heels up as your arms and body are lenghening upward and stay there for 3 seconds (Figure 4-8). Your arms move to open position to move down in front, as the body continues to sink downward (Figure 4-9), then your wrist accrosed in the front of you, both palms facing towards yourself as you exhale (Figure

4-10). When you take your next inhale, your hands and body rise upward, all the joints of the body join the breathing in an expanding motion, and your hands line up with the level of the hight of BL1 points at the inner side of the corner of the eyes (Figure 4-11). Then, open both arms to the side as the arms move downward with palms facing downward with an exhale (Figure 4-12). Don't forget to coordinate all joints of the body in a gentle motion of compressing and relaxing until palms/arms reach their natural positions. Practice 9 repeatations.

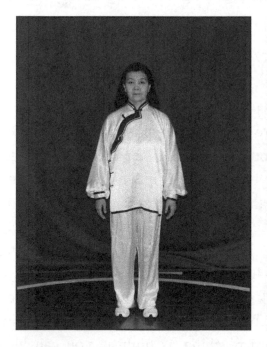
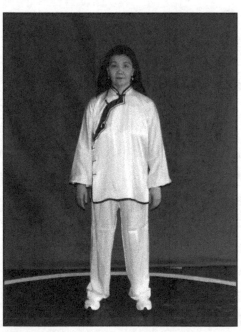

Figure 4-1   Figure 4-2

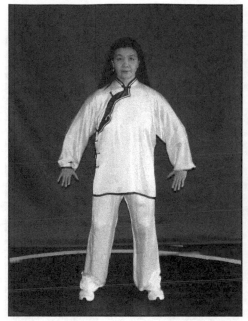

Figure 4-3

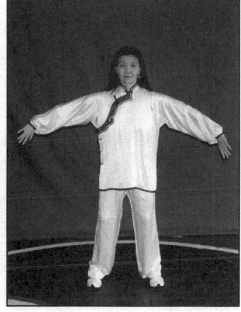

Figure 4-4

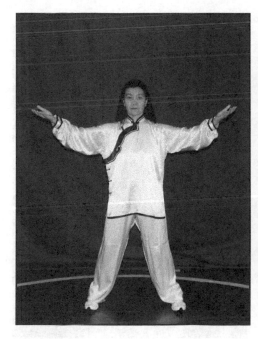

Figure 4-5

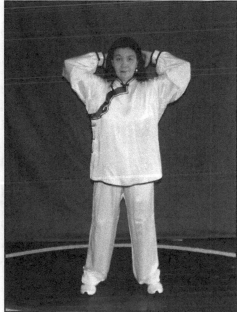

Figure 4-6

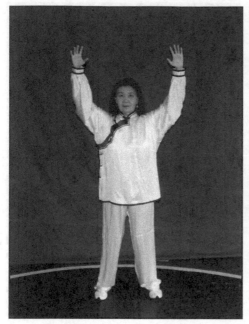

Figure 4-7

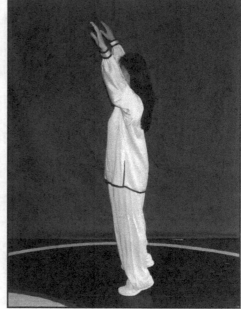

Figure 4-8

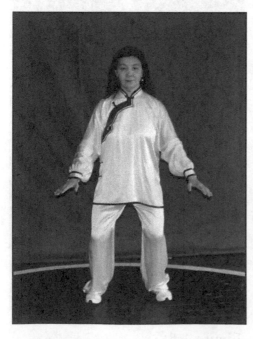

Figure 4-9

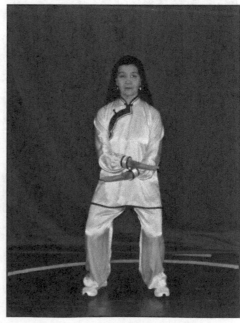

Figure 4-10

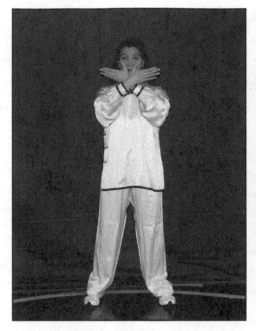

Figure 4-11

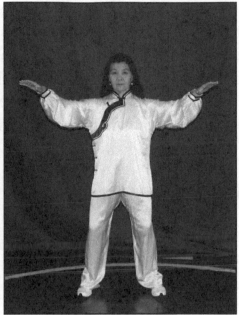

Figure 4-12

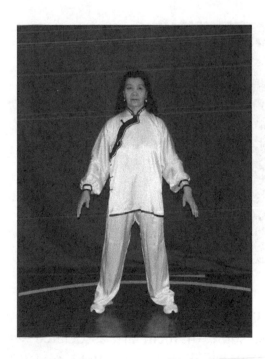

Figure 4-13

The Important Points on Practicing the Physical Movements:
a. Breath naturally and deeply. When you coordinate the movements with inhaling and exhaling, an inhale goes with upwards, outward movements, and an exhale goes with downward, inwards movements.
b. Body motion: always move the entire body at the same time, no individual part of the body moves independently.

2. Connecting to the Universe 自然

Meridian study:
Bladder meridian: this study focuses on the important parts of the Bladder meridian.
Health benefit:
Making more active the back of the body, and help to heal the organs related diseases.

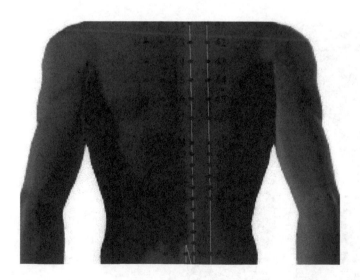

These important points on BL meridian are connecting and transport energy to associated internal organs, some of them are associated with Chinese medicine's anatomical entities. They are from BL13 to BL28, their point names all end with "Shu", meaning transportation in Chinese medicine. Classically, Qi Gong or TCM practitioners try to stimulate these points for the general health of the organs.

There is a total of 16 "Shu" points on the Bladder meridian and they are located about one inch on either side of the spine, from below the third vertebra to below the nineteenth vertebra.

BL13 • Fei Shu 肺俞 (lung)

BL14 • Jue Yin Shu 厥阴俞 (pericardium)

BL15 • Xin Shu 心俞 (heart)

BL16 • Du Shu 督俞 (du, governing channel)

BL17 • Ge Shu 膈俞 (diaphragm)

BL18 • Gan Shu 肝俞 (liver)

BL19 • Dan Shu 胆俞 (gallbladder)

BL20 • Pi Shu 脾俞 (spleen)

BL21 • Wei Shu 胃俞 (stomach)

BL22 • San Jiao Shu 三焦俞 (triple burner)

BL23 • Shen Shu 肾俞 (kidney)

BL24 • Qi Hai Shu 气海俞 (sea of Qi - it's located directly opposite to Sea of Qi (CV6)

BL25 • Da Chang Shu 大肠俞 (large intestine)

BL26 • Guan Yuan Shu 关元俞 (origin pass - it's located directly opposite to origin pass (CV4)

BL27 • Xiao Chang Shu 小肠俞 (small intestine)

BL28 • Pang Guang Shu 膀胱俞 (bladder)

Qi and Meridian

The Yellow Emperor Classic says: "The theory of the five organs and six the Functions do not individually exist. They are all connected and function as a system that works through the network of the meridians to support life."

These acupuncture points relate to all the organs in the body, and some are related to the important Qi points. Some of them are located in relatively the same spots as their corresponding organs, such as heart and lungs, while some of them are not at the same spots with their corresponding organs. Therefore, the Chinese medicine believes these points are transporting the energy to their corresponding organs, and they have been used clinically for balancing the imbalances in these organs, or treating deficiencies in the function of these organs. However, the area between the thoracic spine to the lumbar spine dominates one's general heath from both the Chinese and Western points of view.

This section of our spine, unfortunately, does not move much in our daily activities, and neither are there any special exercises specifically for this section of the spine. The less active part of the body easily becomes a weaker, inflexible part of the body, where the energy decreases and diseases often snake in. Regular Qi Gong exercises and massages to this part of the body can give the internal organs a hand. This is because the Qi Gong motions are gentle, flows the energy to ease the physical pain in this area. Frequently doing it, will benefits the health of both old and young, the ill and the healthy, the martial artists and TCM practitioners themselves.

Qi Gong Movements:
2. Connecting to the Universe (Heaven 2 of 3)

Feet parallel, and apart, at least as the same width of the shoulders or hips; or make the stance a little wider as long as you feel it is comfortable to handle. Your right hand on the Dan Tian, the left arm opens up on the left side (Figure 4-14), start to turn and twist the body to the right side, while the left hand/arm follows the direction that the body is turning to the right with inhale (Figure 4-15); then the left hand pulls inward toward your lower Dan Tian with exhale (Figure 4-16); while the right hand start to swing around with the turning and twisting of the body toward the left side with inhale (Figure 4-17), then reverse the movements and with exhale. These Qi Gong motions work on stimulating and activating these important acupuncture points from the middle to lower back. This is also a fine way to massage the Yang channel.

The movement has to be flowing, while gathering energy from the universe, from our nature surroundings, and from all directions to receive the energy and live with the nature. You will have choices to practice without coordinating breathing; so, the movement speed can be set at three different paces; you can do the exercises three times slowly, then, three times mid speed, and then, three times at a faster speed. You also can set the width of the stance from a shoulder's width stance to a standard horse stance range, or anywhere in between, whatever your own comfort zone is. The weight naturally shifts from side to side, gradually to increase the range of motion around the waist and back. Practice 9 times on each side.

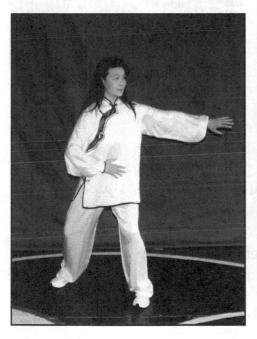 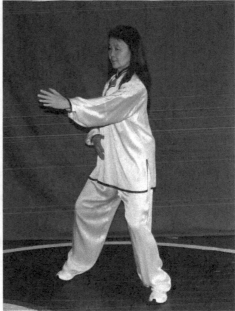

Figure 4-14   Figure 4-15

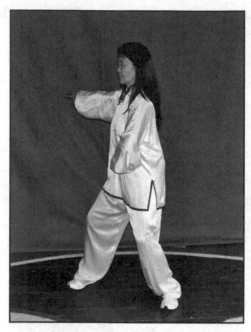
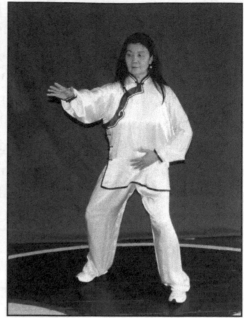

Figure 4-16   Figure 4-17

Important points on practicing the physical movements:
a. The body twists in your natural ability. Breathing is naturally deep.
b. When the movement ends on each side, the hip joints and lower back are loose.
c. One of the beauty of the Qi Gong practice is to start with one's own natural physical abilities and comfortably learning and practicing without forcing to much in physical.

3. Opening the Heart 畅心

Meridian study:

Large Intestine meridian, LI 手阳明大肠经

Heart meridian, HT 手少阴心经

Pericardium meridian, PC 手厥阴心包经

Health benefit:

Good for maintaining heart health.

Large Intestine Meridian - LI - from index finger to underneath of the nose. There are 20 acupuncture points of this meridian.

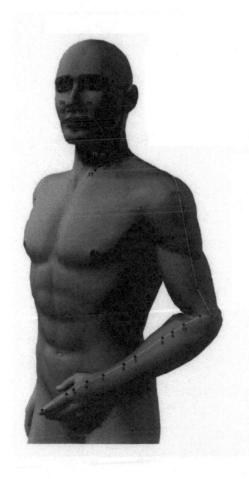

LI - Large Intestine 手阳明大肠经

LI1 • Shang Yang 商阳

LI2 • Er Jian 二间

LI3 • San Jian 三间

LI4 • He Gu 合谷

LI5 • Yang Xi 阳溪

LI6 • Pian Li 偏历

LI7 • Wen Liu 温溜

LI8 • Xia Lian 下廉

LI9 • Shang Lian 上廉

LI10 • Shou San Li 手三里

LI11 • Qu Chi 曲池

LI12 • Zhou Liao 肘廖

LI13 • Shou Wu Li 手五里

LI14 • Bi Nao 臂濡

LI15 • Jian Yu 肩禺

LI16 • Ju Gu 巨骨

LI17 • Tian Ding 天鼎

LI18 • Fu Tu 扶突

LI19 • He Liao 禾廖

LI20 • Ying Xiang 迎香

Heart Meridian, HT, starts from arm pit through the little finger. There are 9 acupuncture points of this meridian.

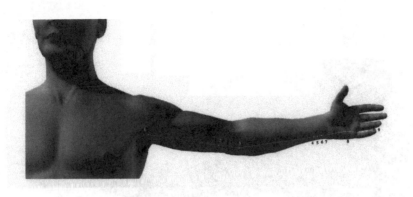

HT - Heart Meridian 手少阴心经
HT1 • Ji Quan 极泉
HT2 • Qing Ling 青灵
HT3 • Shao Hai 少海
HT4 • Ling Dao 灵道
HT5 • Tong Li 通里
HT6 • Yin Xi 阴郄
HT7 • Shen Men 神门
HT8 • Shao Fu 少府
HT9 • Shao Chong 少冲

Pericardium Meridian, PC, is from side of the nipple along the center line of the arm, down to the tip of the middle finger. There are 9 acupuncture points of this meridian.

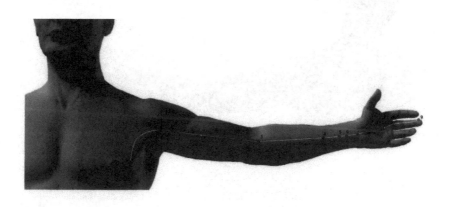

PC - Pericardium Meridian 手厥阴心包经
PC1 • Tian Chi 天池
PC2 • Tian Quan 天泉
PC3 • Qu Ze 曲泽
PC4 • Xi Men 郄门
PC5 • Jian Shi 间使
PC6 • Nei Guan 内关
PC7 • Da Ling 大陵
PC8 • Lao Gong 劳宫
PC9 • Zhong Chong 中冲

Qi and Meridian:

The Yellow Emperor's Classic says: "When the large intestine meridian is full with Qi and blood, it nourishes the Yang energy."

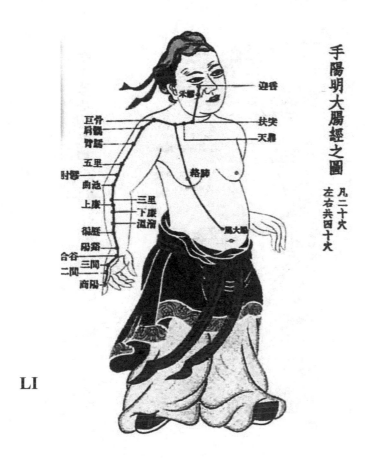

LI

The Large Intestine Meridian, LI, is the reflection of problems relating to the organ. If the body's digestion system is working well, it protects the person from the illness. The energy of the LI meridian working with the body's systems, is an indication to how healthy and flow of the energy in conjunction with the intake and output of nutrition of the body. In other words, if a person has problems with digestion, the symptom of constipation might not only be in the intestines， but may also manifest as problems of the eyes, teeth, acne, nose bleeding and, in many cases, skin problems on the arms, etc. By working on Qi Gong exercises that give the balance back through eliminating toxins, and preventing overheated energy in the body that disturb the functions of the digestion, one can regain their digestive health.

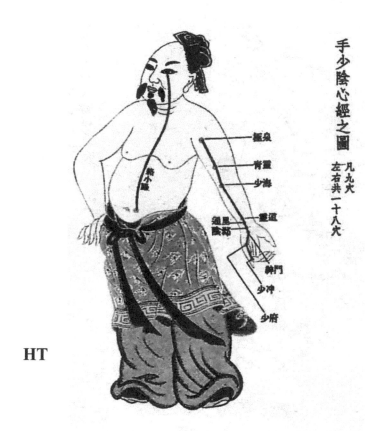

HT

The Yellow Emperor's Classic says: "If the heart is pure and clear, longevity can be achieved; if the heart is out of balance the mind and the body will both be in a dangerous state."

The Heart Meridian, HT, is deeply related to the "Heart" in Chinese worthy beliefs, Heart means spirit, soul, and mind. So exercises for the heart meridian are also to gain a healthy mind and to help the memory, relieve anxiety, sleeplessness, and psychological issues. It is the meridian close to the pericardium meridian so work on both of them together to gain the maxim benefits in heart health.

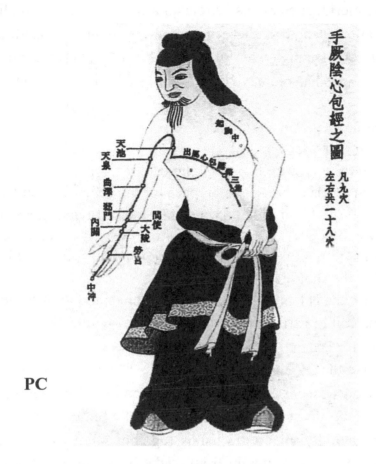

PC

The Pericardium Meridian, PC, is directly related to the health of the heart.

The beginning of the meridian starts with the point "Heaven Pool", traveling all the way through the center of the palm before reaching its end at the tip of the middle finger. The point in the center of the palm PC8劳宫, is known for more than its medical ability, it always has some motions that make a sign of one's happiness, success, cheerfulness, a way to discourage weakness. A natural positivity is defiantly found in our palms! In this segment of Qi Gong, we focus on these three meridians together to strength the heart, and make it stronger in all of its aspects. Another way to look at these three channels is that they relate to the early symptoms of the heart disease or a heart attack. They have commonly been used to sense or realized an attack at the first sign of a heart problem, such as the feeling of pain in these meridian channels or related areas. We need to realize that it is so important to lengthen these meridians by gently expanding arms according your own feelings and abilities within the Qi Gong movement, that enable these meridians to have better blood and Qi circulation.

Qi Gong Movements:
3. Opening the Heart (Heaven 3 of 3)

Before starting, you will be delighted to do some sensing of these three meridian channels exercises to prepare for the efficient results.

1. Exercise the LI meridian: your both index fingers goes outward and forward with the arms lifted to a position just right underneath the nose, then, the index fingers lead the arms open to both sides and keep on the same level of the shoulders.

2. Exercise the HT meridian: open the palms and the little fingers of your both hands coil inward and upward to feel the connection of the little fingers to the armpits.

3. Exercise the PC meridian: both arms stretch out to the side and shifted body weight from side to side to increase the feeling of the connection from outside of the nipples to the middle fingers.

Starting naturally, place the hands together palm to palm (Figure 4-18). Open and close the hands in front of the heart coordinated with the breathing. When the hands open to shoulder's width, inhale. When closing to face's width, exhale (Figure 4-19, 4-20). Then, loosen the hips and sink the center gravity and body weight onto the left leg (Figure 4-21), the right foot steps out to the right side with heel touching the ground first (Figure 4-22), then, shifting 70% of the body weight to the right leg, as the body leans to the right side, while opening the arms and hands with palms facing outwards, look at unweighted leg. Stay for 3 seconds. (Figure 4-23), then, shift the body weight from the right side back towards the right side (Figure 4-24). In other words, returning into the starting position as well as bringing the hands in front of the body about face width, finger tips facing upward., palm to palm (Figure 4-25). Then, repeat on the left side (Figure 4-26, to Figure 4-31). Practice 3 times on each side.

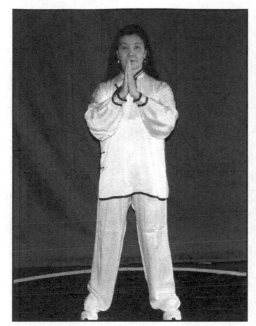

Figure 4-18

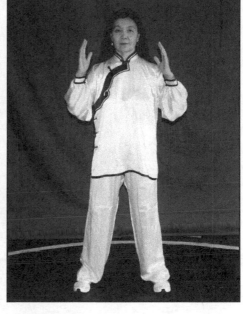

Figure 4-19

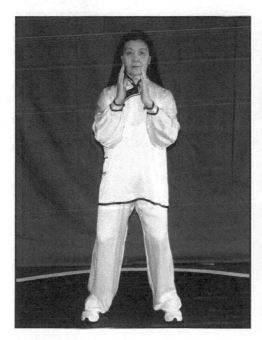

Figure 4-20

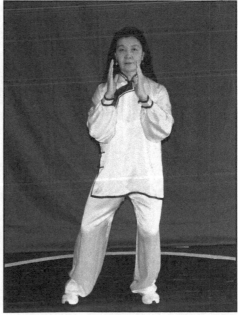

Figure 4-21

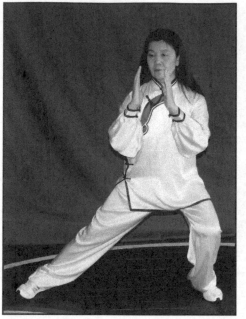

Figure 4-22

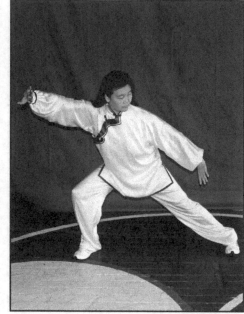

Figure 4-23

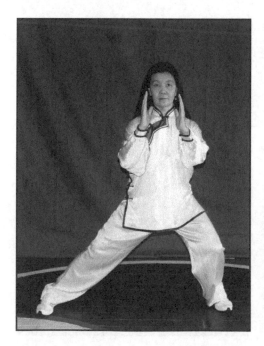

Figure 4-24

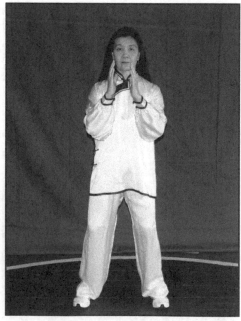

Figure 4-25

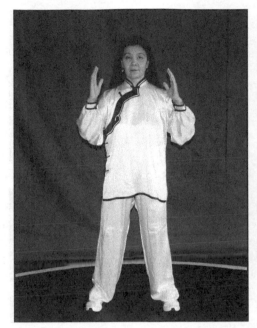

Figure 4-26

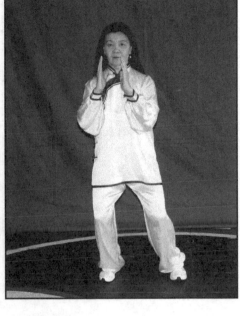

Figure 4-27

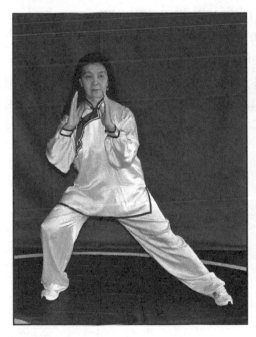

Figure 4-28

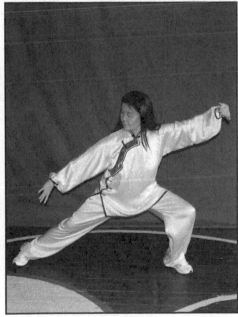

Figure 4-29

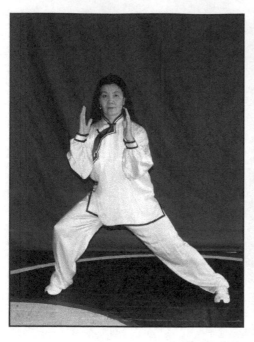 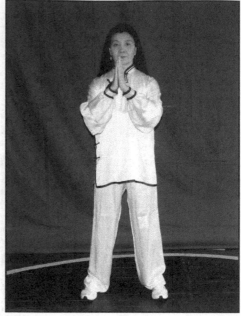

Figure 4-30   Figure 4-31

Important points on practicing the physical movements:
a. The three breathing cycles coordinate with the full body motion.
b. When the body weight shifts, it should be in a gentle manner.
c. The movements that stretch the muscles, tendons, as well as generate the energy of the meridian channels should be at a comfortable levels to each individual's physical ability.

Earth

The Yellow Emperor's Classic says: "Earth provides its Yin energy supporting our lives."

"Water nurtures everything without trying." - Dao De Jing

Earth, our home planet, is a beautiful place to live. Earth is the only planet we know, so far, that can support life, having an abundance of flowing water which provides the essence for all types of life. Beautiful landscapes comprises the visible dynamic features of areas on each part of the earth - there are areas where water and mountains naturally balance the physical elements of Yin and Yang on the land, combined with human elements and creativity make living on the earth an experience of incredible character and quality.

Earth's substantial atmosphere and its magnetic power are critical for continuous biogeochemical cycles, the landscape provides us is why we all live on Earth, not on any other planets, as do other living things: plants, animals, even bacteria. We also easily interact with each other, pleasing each other, and we all have a satisfactory way of our own lives. Earth and all living things are always exchanging energies: The Earth make the soil and water available, human take the energy and are responsible for their environment.

The Earth provides the energy and water makes the energy flow. Through it cycles water travels between different areas of the Earth and about 70% of the Earth's surface is covered with water, most of which consists of the oceans. Only a small portion of the Earth's water is the freshwater, found in rivers, lakes, and groundwater. Freshwater is valuable to human life as it is needed for drinking, farming, and washing, etc. Without water, life as we know it would not exist. It is not our imagination, but a truth that our bodies, just like the Earth, about 60 - 70% of the body is water, that flowing and circulating through the body, supporting the basic needs of life. Water is helping to keep up the body's energy supply, get rid of the wastes, grow and develop. The positive Qi in our body is like water that nurtures everything without tiring. Its power cleans away wastes and purifies the pollutants. Its pureness nourishes the flow of thought and motion.

Our body is like the Earth, it's not healthy if some parts are too dry, too wet, too hot, too cold, and not natural. We need to be balanced to feel comfortable. The Earth's energy is associated to the body's Yin energy, especially those meridians related to the heart, lung, kidney, liver, and spleen. They support the functions of the organs. Nurturing and balance the energy of these meridians helps the internal organs and blood circulation throughout the body.

1. Balancing the Energy 舒中

Meridian study:
Kidney meridian, KI 足少阴肾经
Triple burner meridian, TB 手少阳三焦经
Spleen meridian, SP 足太阴脾经
Stomach meridian, ST 足阳明胃经
Health benefits: Helps to absorb nutritions, clean the system, nurture the internal organs, and physically strengthen the entire body to awaken the internal healing power.

Kidney Meridian, LI, starts from the bottom of the foot along inside of the leg, then, up along the side of the middle line of the body to the upper chest. There are 27 acupuncture points of this meridian.

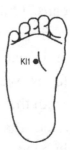

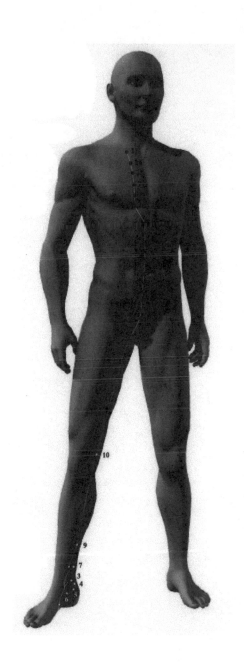

KI - Kidney Meridian 足少阴肾经

KI1 • Yong Quan 涌泉

KI2 • Ran Gu 然谷

KI3 • Tai Xi 太溪

KI4 • Da Zhong 大钟

KI5 • Shui Quan 水泉

KI6 • Zhao Hai 照海

KI7 • Fu Liu 复溜

KI8 • Jiao Xin 交信

KI9 • Zhu Bin 筑宾

KI10 • Yin Gu 阴谷

KI11 • Heng Gu 横骨

KI12 • Da He 大赫

KI13 • Qi Xue 气穴

KI14 • Si Man 四满

KI15 • Zhong Zhu 中注

KI16 • Huan Shu 肓俞

KI17 • Shang Qu 商曲

KI18 • Shi Guan 石关

KI19 • Yin Du 阴都

KI20 • Tong Gu 腹通谷

KI21 • You Men 幽门

KI22 • Bu Lang 步廊

KI23 • Shen Feng 神封

KI24 • Ling Xu 灵墟

KI25 • Shen Cang 神藏

KI26 • Yu Zhong 彧中

KI27 • Shu Fu 俞府

Triple Burner Meridian, TB (or SJ), starts from the ring finger up to the shoulder region, then, right along the border of the ear, ends on the out side of the eyebrow. There are 23 acupuncture points of this meridian.

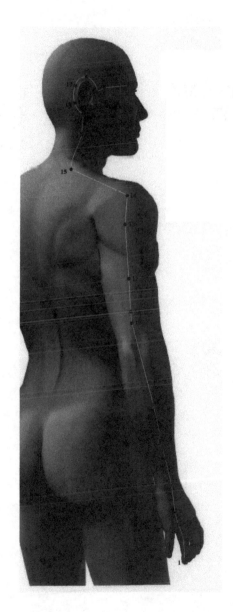

TB - Triple Burner 手少阳三焦经
TB1 • Guan Chong 关冲
TB2 • Ye Men 液门

TB3 • Zhong Zhu 中渚

TB4 • Yang Chi 阳池

TB5 • Wai Guan 外关

TB6 • Zhi Gou 支沟

TB7 • Hui Zong 会宗

TB8 • San Yang Luo 三阳络

TB9 • Si Du 四渎

TB10 • Tian Jing 天井

TB11 • Qing Leng Yuan 清冷渊

TB12 • Xiao Luo 消泺

TB13 • Ru Hui 儒会

TB14 • Jian Liao 肩蓼

TB15 • Tian Liao 天髎

TB16 • Tian You 天牖

TB17 • Yi Feng 翳风

TB18 • Qi Mai 崎脉

TB19 • Lu Xi 颅息

TB20 • Jiao Sun 角孙

TB21 • Er Men 耳门

TB22 • Er He Liao 耳和髎

TB23 • Si Zhu Kong 丝竹空

Spleen Meridian, SP, starts from the inner side of the big toe up to the inguinal region, and up to the side of the chest, and down to the eleventh rib. There are 21 acupuncture points of this meridian.

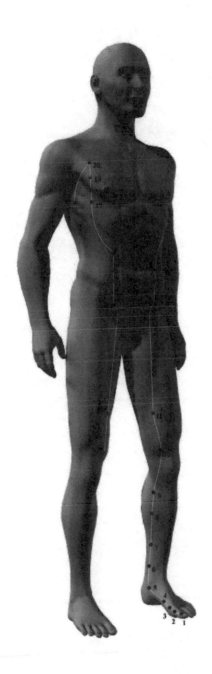

SP - Spleen Meridian 足太阴脾经

SP1 • Yin Bai 隐白

SP2 • Da Du 大都

SP3 • Tai Bai 太白

SP4 • Gong Sun 公孙

SP5 • Shang Qui 商丘

SP6 • San Yin Jiao 三阴交

SP7 • Lou Gu 漏谷

SP8 • Di Ji 地机

SP9 • Yin Ling Quan 阴陵泉

SP10 • Xue Hai 血海

SP11 • Ji Men 箕门

SP12 • Chong Men 冲门

SP13 • Fu She 府舍

SP14 • Fu Jie 腹结

SP15 • Da Heng 大横

SP16 • Fu Ai 腹衰

SP17 • Shi Dou 食窦

SP18 • Tian Xi 天溪

SP19 • Xiong Xiang 胸乡

SP20 • Zhou Rong 周荣

SP21 • Da Bao 大包

Stomach Meridian, ST, Start from right below the center of the eyes down the corners of the mouth, then up to the hair line then, down long the body, after passing through the center of the nipple, it goes close to the center of the body, and all the way down in a little curved line down to the second toe. There are 45 acupuncture points of this meridian.

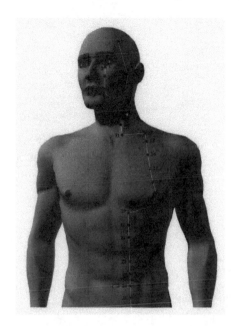

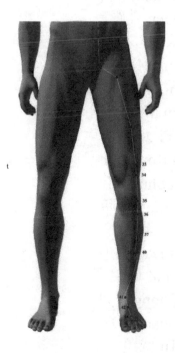

ST - Stomach Meridian 足阳明胃经
ST1 • Cheng Qi 承泣

ST2 • Si Bai 四白
ST3 • Ju Liao 巨廖
ST4 • Di Cang 地仓
ST5 • Da Ying 大迎
ST6 • Jia Che 颊车
ST7 • Xia Guan 下关
ST8 • Tou Wei 头维
ST9 • Ren Ying 人迎
ST10 • Shui Tu 水突
ST11 • Qi She 气舍
ST12 • Que Pen 缺盆
ST13 • Qi Hu 奇户
ST14 • Ku Fang 库房
ST15 • Wu Yi 屋翳
ST16 • Ying Chuang 鹰窗
ST17 • Ru Zhong 乳中
ST18 • Ru Gen 乳跟
ST19 • Bu Rong 不容
ST20 • Cheng Man 承满
ST21 • Liang Men 梁门
ST22 • Guan Men 关门
ST23 • Tai Yi 太乙
ST24 • Hua Rou Men 滑肉门
ST25 • Tian Shu 天枢
ST26 • Wai Ling 外陵
ST27 • Da Ju 大巨
ST28 • Shui Dao 水道
ST29 • Gui Lai 归来
ST30 • Qi Chong 气冲
ST31 • Bi Guan 髀关
ST32 • Fu Tu 伏兔
ST33 • Yin Shi 阴市
ST34 • Liang Qiu 梁丘

ST35 • Du Bi 犊鼻

ST36 • Zu San Li 足三里

ST37 • Shang Ju Xu 上巨虚

ST38 • Tiao Kou 条口

ST39 • Xia Ju Xu 下巨虚

ST40 • Feng Long 丰隆

ST41 • Jie Xi 解溪

ST42 • Chong Yang 冲阳

ST43 • Xian Gu 陷谷

ST44 • Nei Ting 内庭

ST45 • Li Dui 厉兑

Qi and Meridian:

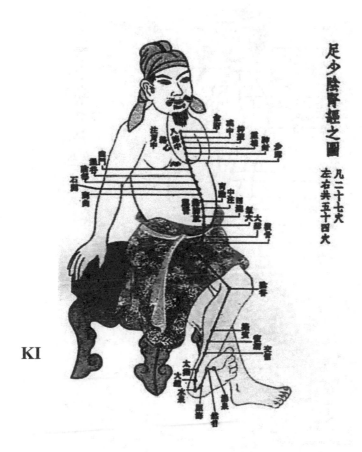

KI

The Kidney Meridian, KI, is a water channel starting from the bottom of the foot, it is as important as water is to life, so the acupuncture point KI1 is referred to as the "Nurturing Life Point." It is also described in Chinese medicine as the "essence" of one's health with its relationship to the kidneys. In other words, the kidneys belong to the water character that holds the source of human being's original development and is the basic element of life. Since this meridian travels through the inner side of the leg and inner side of the body, which connect the most organs, many medical problems are related to a weakness in the kidneys, including fertility problems and disorders of the sexual energy.

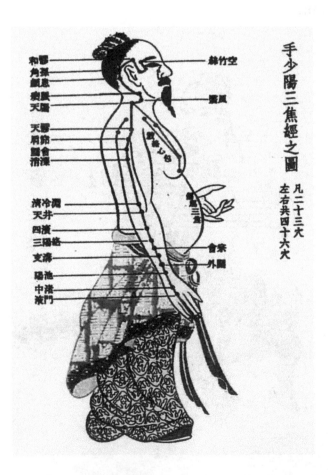

TB

The Triple Burners Meridian, TB, is a quiet agent that takes care of the triple burners.

The triple burner is not an organ, it acts like a container that holds the trunk of upper body. Chinese medicine separates the internal upper body into three parts, according the organs. The upper burner includes heart and lungs, middle burner is below the diaphragm including the stomach and the spleen; and below the naval is the lower burner where the kidneys, bladder, large and small intestines are. The meridian is on the outside of the arm around the ear area, but like all the meridians that have inner connections, the triple burner channels treat all Qi, energy related, chronic diseases or disorders that come from inside the body. You may realize that, any health problem shown externally, has a source of the problem on the inside. It's a part of understanding traditional Chinese medicine on how it looks at the entire body as a whole and only sees localized symptoms, but not localized diseases. Health promotion in Chinese medicine is built on the principle of the unity of human beings.

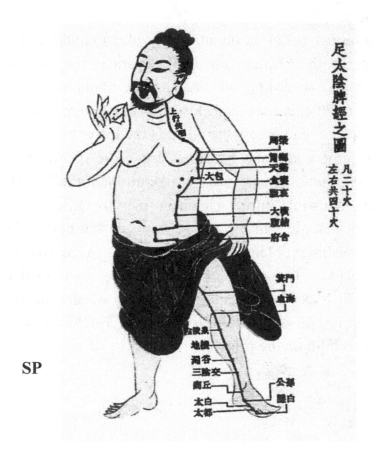

SP

The Spleen Meridian, SP, is a special agent of the body. The functions of this meridian are a little differently defined than the functions of the anatomical spleen. In Chinese medicine view, the spleen meridian is expected to balance the Qi and blood through the inner side of the body and to help the circulation passing through the inguinal region. It helps to balance a lacking of Yin energy. Since it connects the three strong Yin meridians of the kidneys, spleen and liver through one important point SP6, this meridian channel is held in great repute as a powerful source of treatments for the reproductive organs. It is especially respected as a help with gynecological problems.

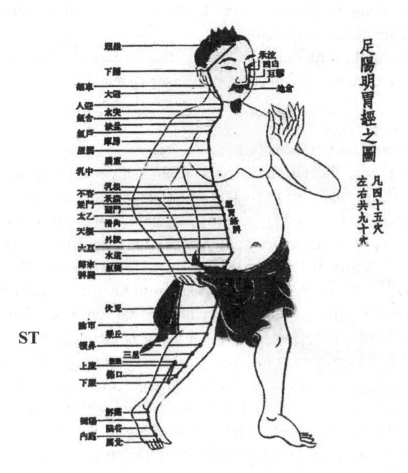

ST

The Stomach Meridian, ST, is another long meridian and passes all the way through the body. It also has many basic energy relationships with the effects of food and many abnormal issues though out the body. A healthy body is not only about what you eat, what to take into the body, but also about how the body can absorb and digest well. Sometimes, digestive problems are the sources of other problems, which becomes a major issue for many people, and many times, the problems are not really localized in the abdominal area. The famous "Longevity Point," ST36, is located below the knee along the channel, and legendarily used by many very respected Chinese doctors to treat many problems in the history of Chinese medicine, including the problems from headaches to digestive issues and anything that annoys one physically.

Exercising these four meridian all together to have two Yin and two yang energy balance to expect a cleaner, stronger system.

Qi Gong Movements:
1. Balancing the Energy (Earth 1 of 3)

Starting with the left foot steps to the left and place the feet paralleled on the ground, about shoulder width or hip width apart, the body weight is centered (Figure 4-32). Forming the "hold ball" position with the left hand on top, palm facing down, the left hand is placed no higher than the neck; the right hand palm faces up, is hold no lower than the Dan Tian (Figure 4-33). Then, the right hand moving upward while the left hand is moving downward. This changes the right hand on top of the left hand (Figure 4-34). Keeps moving upward, the palm is facing forward while the left hand moving down to the front of the abdomen, the palm facing downward, both hands should be staying in front of the body (Figure 4-35). Then, bend forward and downward with entire spine gently expanded motion (Figure 4-36), after you reaching to the point that you feel comfortably stretched, twisting the body to the left side (Figure 4-37), and straightening back up to the standing position, without changing either of the hand's position (Figure 4-38). Then, shift body weight to the left side (Figure 4-39). Start with the right hand pulling backward till the palm faces the right ear, strengthening through the ring fingers; simultaneously, the left hand is reaching the direction towards the right heel while the right leg lifts up with the right keen slightly pointing towards right side, for opening the inner side of the legs and help more blood circulates throughout the inner side of leg. At the same time, the right heel is pushing forward gently (Figure 4-40). Then, step the right foot backward with a small step while both palms facing downward (Figure 4-41); then the left foot steps back and paralleled with right foot at shoulder width (Figure 4-42). Repeat on the right side (Figure 4-43 to Figure 4-51). Practice 3 times on each side.

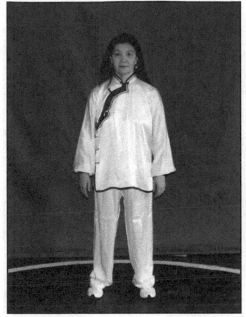

Figure 4-32

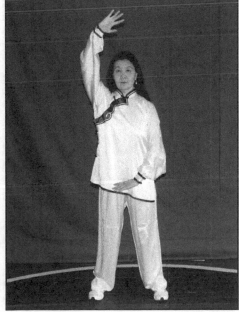

Figure 4-33

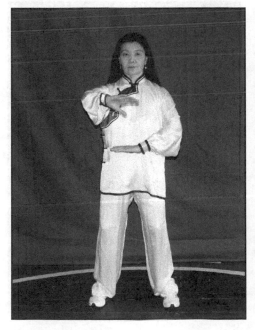

Figure 4-34

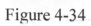

Figure 4-35

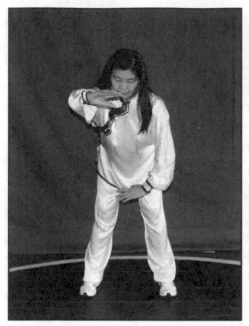

Figure 4-36

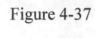

Figure 4-37

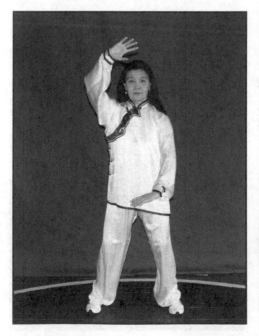

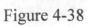

Figure 4-38

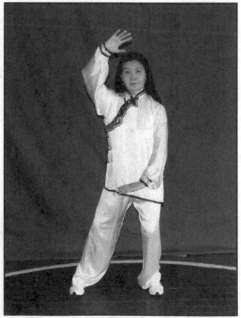

Figure 4-39

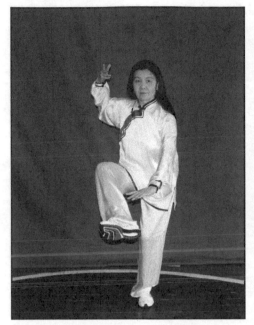

Figure 4-40

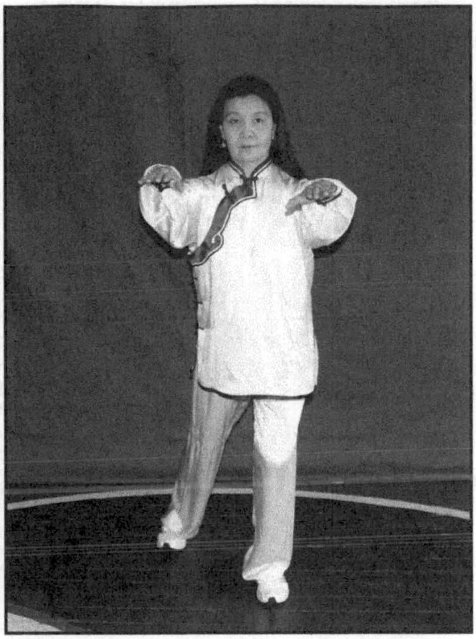

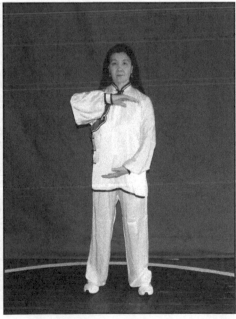

Figure 4-41

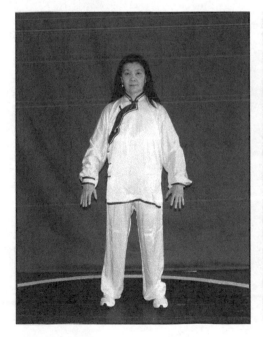

Figure 4-42

Figure 4-43

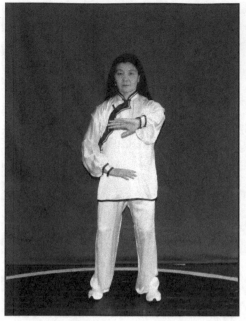

Figure 4-44

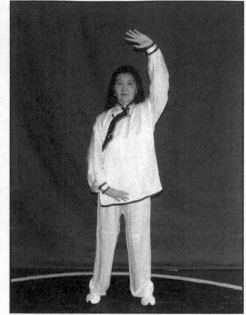

Figure 4-45

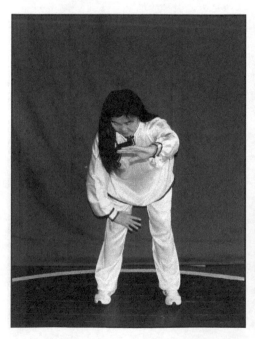

Figure 4-46

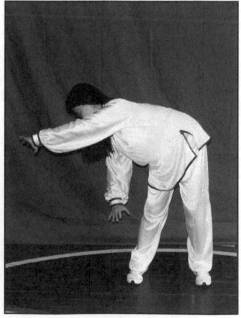

Figure 4-47

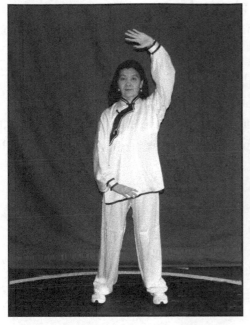

Figure 4-48

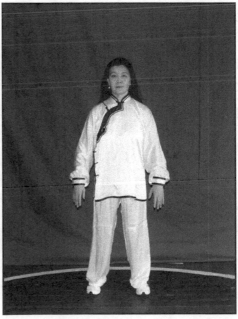

Figure 4-49

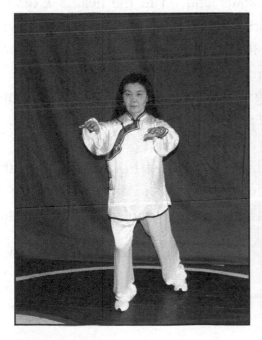

Figure 4-50

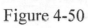

Figure 4-51

Important points on practicing the physical movements:

a. You do what you feel natural and comfortable when bend the body forward and downward.

b. When step back, take a small step that you can physically feel still in balance.

c. This section involves four meridians study and relatively complicated physical motion. The coordination and balance of the movements will also be strongly trained and practiced.

2. Strengthen the Essentials 强体

Meridian study:

Liver meridian LV, 足厥阴肝经

Gallbladder meridian GB, 足少阳胆经

Health benefit: One yin and one yang meridian, the liver meridian starts from the foot and runs to the gallbladder and on to the head. Exercise them together to help the body absorb nutrition properly. This also works on balancing the emotions, easing the feelings of any displeasure, and releasing physical exhaustion. Research has shown that strengthening these meridians is a unique way of helping to heal some neurological problems, especially around the legs and sciatic nerves.

Liver Meridian, LV, start from the inner side of the big toe, up along the inner side of the leg to the pubic region, then, cross to the opposite side of the body and end below the nipple. There are14 acupuncture points of this meridian.

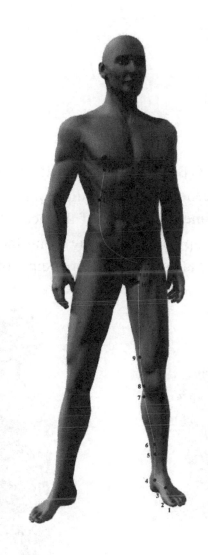

LV - Liver Meridian 足厥阴肝经

LV1 • Da Dun 大敦

LV2 • Xing Jian 行间

LV3 • Tai Chong 太冲

LV4 • Zhong Feng 中封

LV5 • Li Gou 蠡沟

LV6 • Zhong Du 中都

LV7 • Xi Guan 膝关

LV8 • Qu Quan 曲泉

LV9 • Yin Bao 阴包

LV10 • Zu Wu Li 足五里
LV11 • Yin Lian 阴廉
LV12 • Ji Mai 急脉
LV13 • Zhang Men 章门
LV14 • Qi Men 期门

Gallbladder Meridian, GB, Start from the outer corner of the eye, around the ear and go to the center above middle point of the eyebrow, travel down through the hair line to the side of the neck, then, down along the side of the body, to the hip and all the way along the outside of the leg to the fourth toe's tip. There are 44 acupuncture points of this meridian.

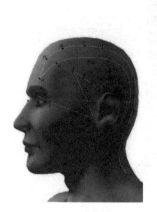

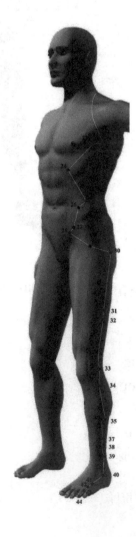

GB - Gallbladder Meridian 足少阳胆经

GB1 • Tong Zi Liao 童子窌

GB2 • Ting Hi 听会

GB3 • Shang Guan 上关

GB4 • Han Yan 颔厌

GB5 • Xuan Lu 悬颅

GB6 • Xuan Li 悬厘

GB7 • Qu Bin 曲鬓

GB8 • Shuai Gu 率谷

GB9 • Tian Chong 天冲

GB10 • Fu Bai 浮白

GB11 • Tou Qiao Yin 头窍阴

GB12 • Wan Gu 完骨

GB13 • Ben Shen 本神

GB14 • Yang Bai 阳白

GB15 • Tou Lin Qi 头临泣

GB16 • Mu Chuang 目窗

GB17 • Zheng Ying 正营

GB18 • Cheng Ling 承灵

GB19 • Nao Kong 脑空

GB20 • Feng Chi 风池

GB21 • Jian Jing 肩井

GB22 • Yuan Ye 渊腋

GB23 • Zhe Jin 辄筋

GB24 • Ri Yue 日月

GB25 • Jing Men 京门

GB26 • Dai Mai 带脉

GB27 • Wu Shu 五枢

GB28 • Wei Dao 维道

GB29 • Ju Liao 居窌

GB30 • Huan Tiao 环跳

GB31 • Feng Shi 风市

GB32 • Zhong Du 中渎

GB33 • Xi Yang Guan 膝阳关

GB34 • Yang Ling Quan 阳陵泉

GB35 • Yang Jiao 阳交

GB36 • Wai Qui 外丘

GB37 • Guang Ming 光明

GB38 • Yang Fu 阳辅

GB39 • Xuan Zhong 悬钟

GB40 • Qiu Xu 丘墟

GB41 • Zu Lin Qi 足临泣

GB42 • Di Wu Hui 地五会

GB43 • Jia Xi 侠溪

GB44 • Zu Qiao Yin 足窍阴

Qi and Meridians:

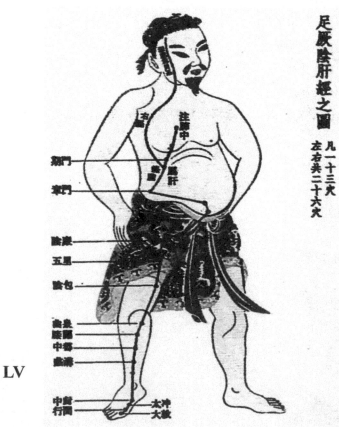

LV

The Liver Meridian, LV, is a commander in the "palace" of the body system, a very important meridian also characterize one's health, also an organ that easily gets attacked, often has its functions weakened by people's life styles. This section of Qi Gong exercise is about using twisting motions to strengthen this meridian, like opening the windows so that the exercise becomes favorable for the organs as a well-known posture, "Breath-in-fresh-air to the body." Lengthening begins at the point LV1 and continues to the ending point LV14. Making more Qi and blood around the pubic area and up to the area below the nipples. It is needlessness to say how much that can benefit internal health and balance emotional "fire" (anger) that comes from a liver function deficiency.

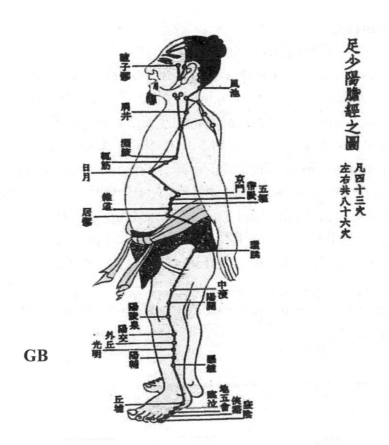

GB

The **Gallbladder Meridian, GB,** is a very important meridian that helps other organs function well. It starts from the side of the eyes, relatively along the side of the head, side of the upper and lower body. There are some points popularly used in acupuncture or massage, such as GB4, GB20, GB21, that help with common colds, headaches and sleeping problems. Practically, this section of Qi Gong twists the body to stimulate the energy to give the internal organs a gentle way of self-massage. My personal clinical experience and research has shown that strengthening these meridians by focusing on the area of the point GB30 makes a unique way of helping to heal some neurological problems, especially around legs and sciatic nerves.

Qi Gong Movement:

2. Strengthening the Essentials (Earth 2 of 3)

Sinking down the center gravity, and the left foot steps straight forward (Figure 4-52), the body weight shifting forward to form a front stance, which is about 70% of the body weight is on the front leg; meanwhile, twist the body from the waist to the left side, the right arm simultaneously moving with the palm facing down about the eye level; while the left palm facing backward and outward, with twisted the body and looking back. The right heel can be lifted up a little bit without touching the ground for your comfort in this twisting position, or, stay on the ground if you are flexible enough (Figure 4-53). Holding this posture about 3 seconds. Then the right foot steps forward to start to repeat the movement you just did on the other side (Figure 5-54, 5-55). Practice 9 times on each side.

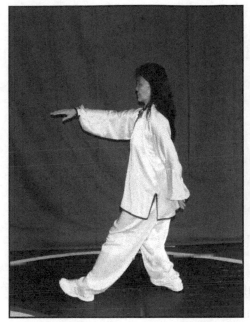

Figure 4-52

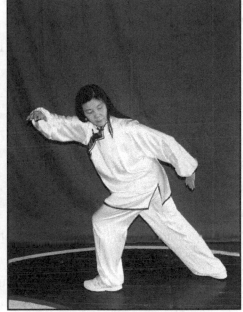

Figure 4-53

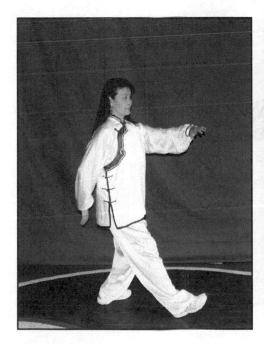

Figure 4-54

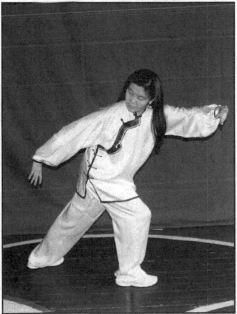

Figure 4-55

Important points on practicing the physical movements:
a. Twist body gently and look back.
b. When the body is twisting, the heel of the back foot can be off the ground for your comfort.

3. Flowing the Earth Energy 坤气

Meridian study:
Lung meridian, LU 手太阴肺经
Health benefits:
Breathing deeply for the Lung's health.

Lung Meridian, LU, start from the upper chest near and above the armpit, travel along the inside of the upper arm down to the thumb. There are 11 acupuncture points of this meridian.

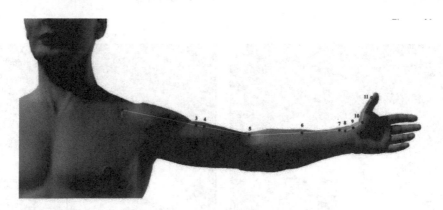

LU - Lung Meridian
LU1 • Zhong Fu 中府
LU2 • Yun Men 云门
LU3 • Tian Fu 天府
LU4 • Xia Bai 侠白
LU5 • Chi Ze 尺泽
LU6 • Kong Zui 孔最
LU7 • Lie Que. 列缺

LU8 • Jing Qu 经渠
LU9 • Tai Yuan 太渊
LU10 • Yu Ji 鱼际
LU11 • Shao Shang 少商

Qi and Meridian:

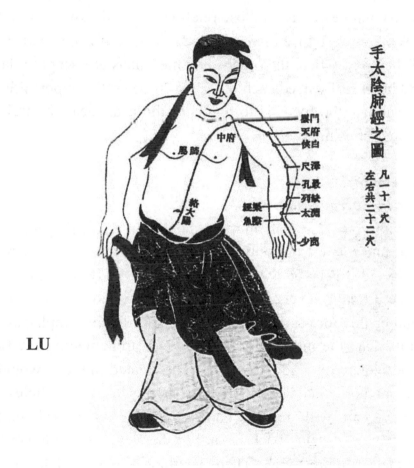

LU

The Lung Meridian, LU, is a big help in preserving the lung's health. Breathing is one of the signature aspects in medical Qi Gong that exercise the lungs and entire chest cavity. Breathing well is not only limited to lung health, but also is a method of emotionally calming down, that easies many excessively excited, or nervous situations in life. The LU1 point is frequently used to directly treat lung problems.

The Yellow Emperor's classic says: "The Lung meridian can tell the manners of all the meridians." It is so considerable to view this meridian as a reflection of one's overall health. Chinese doctors pulse the LU7 and LU8 points in this area to check out their patient's general health. Commonly, the Lung meridian is the first meridian to be introduced to people who are interested in studying Chinese medicine.

The lungs and heart have a close relationship to the over all system of the body. When we exercise the lungs, we also exercise the heart in the same area of the body, where the organs and meridians are deeply related. The lungs and heart really need each other's well being to support life. In this Qi Gong section, the focus is to regulates the heart beats by training the longer, deeper breathing.

Qi Gong Movement:
3. Flowing Earth Energy (Earth 3 of 3)

Stand with your feet apart in your shoulder's width (Figure 4-56). Both arms coil and rotate from outward (Figure 4-57) to inward, circling around from the side of the body to the center of the body with the thumb leading in three different levels. Because the Lung meridian end near the tip of the thumb, this movement of Qi Gong specifically emphases and uses the thumbs lead the motion for opening up, strengthening the Lung area of the body internally and externally. The rotated motions would be in three different horizontal levels, in three complete deep inhales and exhales. First, start with natural hands pressing downward, coiling outward while inhale, circling back inward to the level of the lower Dan Tian while exhale (Figure 4-58). Then, continue the second level with hands and arms coiling outwards while inhale (Figure 4-59), circling back in, towards chest level while exhale (Figure 4-60). Then, continues the arms reach higher up while inhale (Figure 4-61, 4-62), and the arms downward while exhale (Figure 4-63). Then repeat 9 times.

Important points on practicing the physical movements:
a. Each horizontal levels of arms movement coordinate one complete breathing with an inhale and exhale. Keep a good pace of breathing.

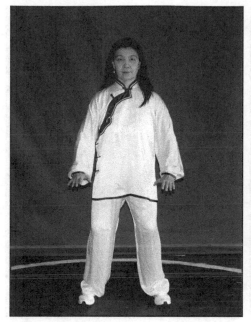

Figure 4-56

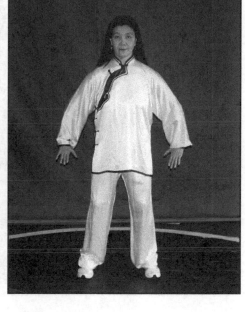

Figure 4-57

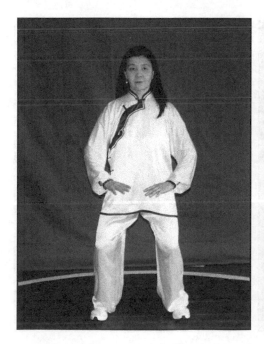

Figure 4-58

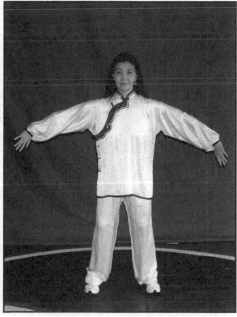

Figure 4-59

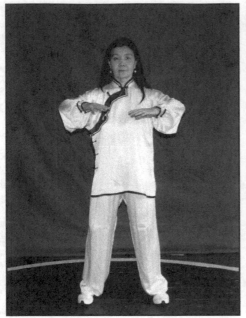

Figure 4-60

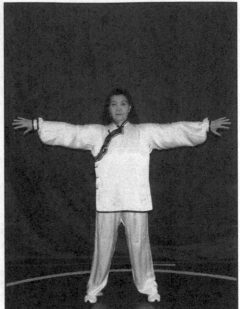

Figure 4-61

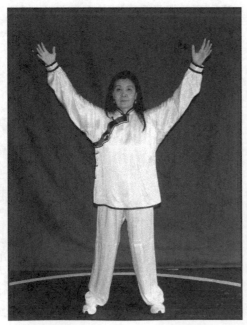

Figure 4-62

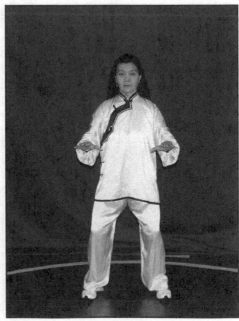

Figure 4-63

Human

"Heaven has laws, and Earth maintains principles. The freedom in between is Human Nature." - Tina Chunna Zhang

The most wonderful creation of Heaven and Earth is human beings! The beauty of being a human is that each of us are always making splendid appearances and having magnificent experiences throughout our fine lives. There are so many words to say about this but the idea can never be fully expressed.

1. Cultivating Energy 补气

Meridian study:
Small Intestine Meridian, SI 手太阳小肠经
Benefit: Complementary for storing energy in Dan Tian and balancing the heart meridian.

Small Intestine, SI, starts at the tip of the little finger and travels up along the back of the arm, curving around the scapular region, and up the neck to the cheek, ending at the pressure point in front of the center of the ear. 19 points.

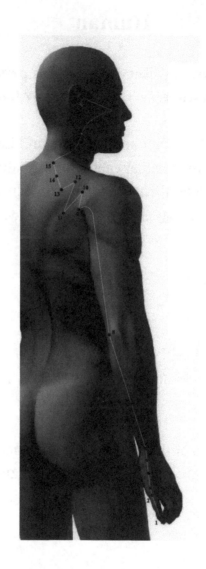

SI - Small Intestine 手太阳小肠经

SI1 • Shao Ze 少泽

SI2 • Qian Gu 前谷

SI3 • Hou Xi 后溪

SI4 • Wan Gu 腕骨

SI5 • Yang Gu 阳谷

SI6 • Yang Lao 养老

SI7 • Zhi Zheng 支正

SI8 • Xiao Hai 小海

SI9 • Jian Zhen 肩贞

SI10 • Nao Shu 需俞

SI11 • Tian Zong 天宗

SI12 • Bing Feng 秉风

SI13 • Qu Yuan 曲垣

SI14 • Jian Wai Shu 肩外俞

SI15 • Jian Zhong Shu 肩外俞

SI16 • Tian Chuang 天窗

SI17 • Tian Rong 天容廖

SI18 • Quan Liao 颧廖

SI19 • Ting Gong 听宫

Qi and Meridian:

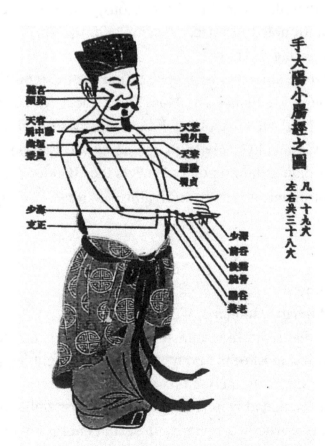

SI

The Small Intestine Meridian, SI, is a complementary channel for storing energy in the Dan Tian. The physical distance of the Small intestine is far away from the SI meridian. The meridian and the organ only connect through their energy pathway and the flow of the blood circulation that reaches the far side of the body, such as the little finger and ear, and then returns to the deepest center of the body. It is also a meridian which reflects heart conditions.

According to the Traditional Chinese Medicine beliefs, the cultivation of a human's essential energy around the Dan Tian area will restore Qi as well as producing an effect of empowering the sexual energy. As the small intestine is in the Dan Tian area, often many problems in the small intestine effect the emotions and disturb mental calmness and contentment. At some point of life, many people have been experienced that emotional disorders can first be obviously seen or feel through the symptoms of a troubled stomach system and the difficulty of storing, diluting, and digesting food.

The Qi Gong movements in this section are the modifications of the Father of Chinese Medicine, Dr. Hua Tuo's Deer Walk from his Five Animal Frolics Medical Qi Gong. Practicing these exercises often will strength one's over all physical health, including the eyes and ears.

This meridian's ending point connects the Bladder meridian through the eyes to communicate with cultivating a greater Yang energy that nurture the Yin energy.

Qi Gong Movement:
1. Cultivating Energy (Human 1 of 3)

Pivoting the right foot into 45 degree angle, the left foot steps forward but bearing most of the body weight on the right leg (Figure 4-64). Both arms come up as the pelvis tilts upward to exercise the external the sexual organs of men, and women. When one gently tightening and lifting their pelvic floors upward that pumps up sexual energy by exercising these physical organs.

Cultivating energy in Qi Gong has a lot to do with the stimulation of these two extraordinary meridians which are Governing and Conception meridians. They are also widely known among the Daoist health practice. The two well-known meridians are vertically located in the center of the upper body, circular the energy between the front and back. This motion focuses on stimulating the areas of the CV1 and GV1 points (Figure 4-65). Then, upward motion is continued to lengthen the spine with a slight lean backwards while the arms come up, high enough that the eyes can see the palms. Meanwhile, the little fingers coiled inward, naturally opening up onto little wider than one's shoulders width. Then, holding this posture exercise the eyes by rotating the eye balls clockwise and then, counter clockwise. Hold the posture in stillness while listening for any sounds coming from one's behind to bring the focus onto the area where the small intestine meridian's ending point SI19, for 3 seconds. When your posture is in stillness, keep the breath of continuousness. This posture is to enable the body's energy coming from the lower Dan Tian and lower back reaches to the crown of the head, around the acupuncture points of GB20. This is also preparing for the next section to harmonize the whole body's energy (Figure 4-66). Then, adjust the body from a slightly leaned back position to a straight position, that enables the top of the head to connect to Heaven by gently lifting the head from the spine and neck to help clarity of the mind, enable the brain to rest (Figure 4-67). When both hands and arms slowly come down (Figure 4-68), the spine is kept straight. The center is aligned while sinking the center of gravity, relaxing the pelvic area to connect to the Earth; the most of the body weight still kept on the right foot - that's how you make more room physically between the legs and thigh, that enable more energy flow in this   area - in front of the anus extending to the couchette of the vulva in the female and to the scrotum in the male. Then, privet left foot in 45 degree angle, the right foot steps straight forward touch the ground, but the body weight is kept on the left foot. Repeat on the this side, a total of 3 times on each side (Figure 4-69 through 4-73). When you finish, steps up into a basic standing posture.

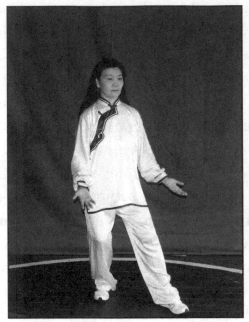

Figure 4-64

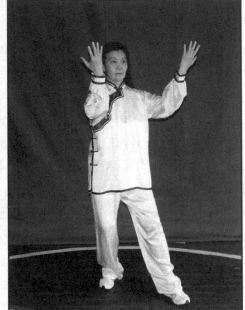

Figure 4-65

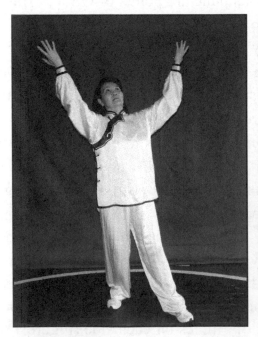

Figure 4-66

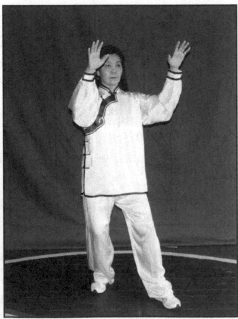

Figure 4-67

131

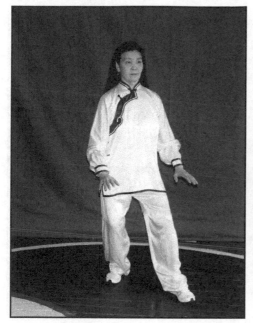

Figure 4-68

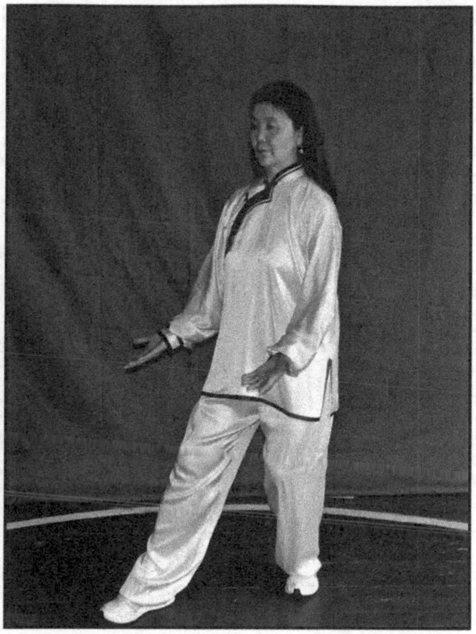

Figure 4-69

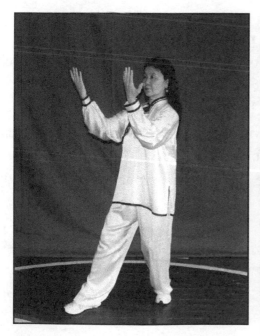

Figure 4-70

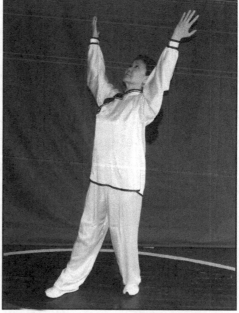

Figure 4-71

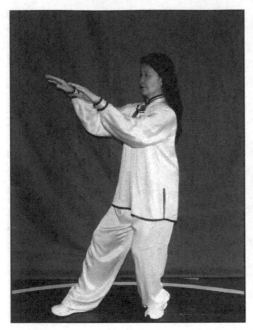 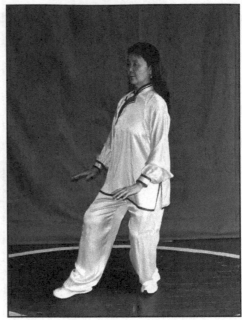

Figure 4-72   Figure 4-73

Important points on practicing the physical movements:
a. When lengthening the spine, do not bent the neck backward too much, keep a natural connection between the spine and head.
b. When circling the eye balls should be gentle, slow, and comfortable.
c. Only need to at take a small step when stepping forward, which you can handle the body weight on the back foot easily.
d. Up to this section, you complete the twelve primary meridian study. Cheers!

2. Harmony of the Three Treasures 和谐

Meridian study:
Governing Vessel meridian (GV, Du) 督脉
Conception Vessel Meridian (CV, Ren) 任脉
Health benefits:
Stimulation of human potential.

The Governing Vessel Meridian, GV, starts midway between the tip of the coccyx bone and the anus. It flows upward inside the spinal column to the nape of the neck, and ascends to the vertex. Along the forehead, it descends to the bridge of the nose , then to the lips. Ending at the labial frenulum inside the upper lip. There are 28 acupuncture points of this meridian.

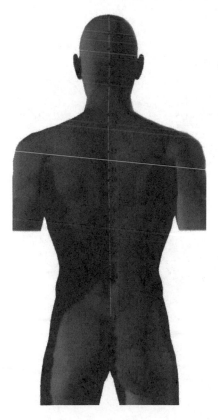

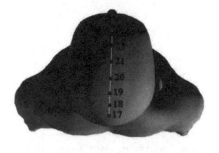 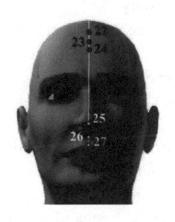

GV - Governing Vessel Meridian 督脉

GV1 • Chang Qiang 长强

GV2 • Yao Shu 腰俞

GV3 • Yao Yang Guan 腰阳关

GV4 • Ming Men 命门

GV5 • Xuan Shu 悬枢

GV6 • Ji Zhong 脊中

GV7 • Zhong Shu 中枢

GV8 • Jin Suo 筋缩

GV9 • Zhi Yang 至阳

GV10 • Ling Tai 灵台

GV11 • Shen Dao 神道

GV12 • Shen Zhu 身柱

GV13 • Tao Dao 陶道

GV14 • Da Zhui 大椎

GV15 • Ya Men 哑门

GV16 • Feng Fu 风府

GV17 • Nao Hu 脑户

GV18 • Qiang Jian 强间

GV19 • Hou Ding 后顶

GV20 • Bai Hi 百会
GV21 • Qian Ding 前顶
GV22 • Xin Hui 囟会
GV23 • Shang Xing 上星
GV24 • Shen Ting 神庭
GV25 • Su Liao 素髎
GV26 • Shui Gou 水沟
GV27 • Dui Duan 兑端
GV28 • Yin Jiao 龈交

The Conception Vessel Meridian, CV, starts on the midline between the anus and the scrotum in males. Between the anus and the posterior labial commissure in females. It ascends anteriorly to the public region. Along the midline of the abdomen, it flows upward till it reaches the throat. Flowing further upward, it ends in the depression in the center of the the groove. There are 24 acupuncture points of this meridian.

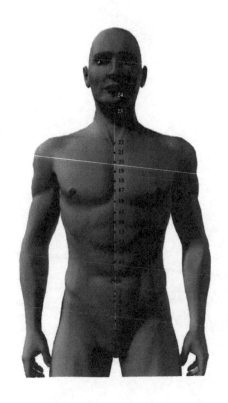

CV - Conception Vessel Meridian 任脉

CV1 • Hui Yin 会阴
CV2 • Qu Gu 曲骨
CV3 • Zhong Ji 中极
CV4 • Guan Yuan 关元
CV5 • Shi Men 关元
CV6 • Qi Hai 气海
CV7 • Yin Jiao 阴交
CV8 • Shen Que 神厥
CV9 • Shui Fen 水分
CV10 • Xia Guan 下脘
CV11 • Jian Li 建里
CV12 • Zhon Guan 中脘
CV13 • Shan Guan 上脘
CV14 • Ju Que. 巨厥
CV15 • Jiu Wei 鸠尾
CV16 • Zhong Ting 中庭
CV17 • Shan Zhong 膻中
CV18 • Yu Tang 玉堂
CV19 • Zi Gong 紫宫
CV20 • Hua Gai 华盖
CV21 • Xuan Ji 璇玑
CV22 • Tian Tu 天突
CV23 • Lian Quan 廉泉
CV24 • Cheng Jiang 承浆

Qi and Meridian:
The Microcosmic Orbit 小周天
The Macrocosmic Orbit 大周天

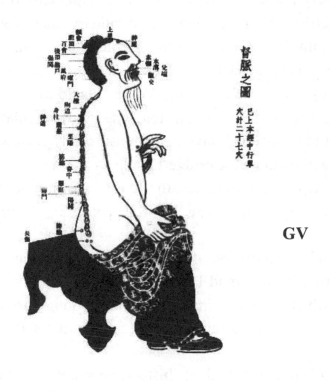

督脈之圖
巳上本經中行畢
大計二十七穴

GV

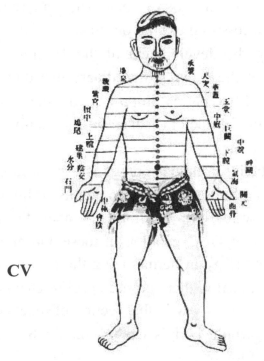

任脈之圖
巳上本經中行畢
大計二十四穴

CV

Beside the twelve primary meridian channels, there are eight extraordinary meridians. The functions of these eight extraordinary meridians are supporting and coordinating the Qi in the primary meridians. Six out of these eight extraordinary meridians have no their own specific points, only two of them have; they are the **Governing Vessel Meridian, GV,** and **Conception Vessel Meridian, CV.** These two meridians circulate and guide the central Qi in the body, and have been considerably reviewed by different groups of practitioners as a bridge that links the Yin and Yang energies in the body. "Opening the access" to the microcosmic orbits is a foremost step in the beginning stage of the process of building extraordinary health.

In Daoist view of Qi circulation of the GV and CV meridians make up the microcosmic orbit, or the Small Heavenly Circle, Xiao Zhou Tian, 小周天 in Chinese, which is most important Daoist and martial arts practice for cultivating of human essence, energy, and spirit for longevity and a good healthy life.

In the legends of Chinese martial arts history, people with extremely high skills were always the one who had removed the blockages and opened the access to their microcosms.

Along the development of the Traditional Chinese Medicine, the importance of these two extraordinary meridians for health is commonly acknowledged to be as important as the primary twelve meridians. Therefore, the fourteen meridians is commonly recognized in the medical practice in China.

The belief in human energy is expressed by the Qi cycle of Heaven and Earth, and builds the treasure quality of human life. In this section of Qi Gong practice, we are not only open the access and establish the fundamentals of Qi circulation in these Yin and Yang channels, but also cultivate the energy in harmonizing the energy of the Heaven, Earth, and Human. Technically, there are no specific channels to always focus on or guiding points to follow in this section of practice; the sensation of natural flow of the whole body's energy should be experienced according the principles of Qi Gong.

We are moving onto the sense of how the power of the three treasures affects each individual, engages, and harmonizes them through the motions of the exercises. As a result, the purpose of the remaining practice in this section is to extend the practice into the Macrocosmic Orbit, Da Zhou Tian, 大周天. Fortunately, we can experience the part of our own energy field which is a circle around each individual. Each person is a microcosm of the universe. This circular energy pattern holds one's central thoughts strongly as being oneself and able to defend or guard one's self from attack, annoyance or insult, and to shield one from injury or danger.

The quality of constancy of Qi circulation in the entire body creates softness in feelings, reduces stagnation in motions, and gradually forms a naturally developed state of mind and body that works with the concept of the three treasures: When the Heaven places greater responsibility on a person and frustrates his or her spirit and will; the Earth will support this person's independency, nurtures his or her body; they form a better being who is free from any influence, negativity, or limitation, and can create his or her own new world!

Qi Gong Movement:
2. Harmony of the Three Treasures (Human 2 of 3)

Stepping the left foot to the left side to form a riding-horse-stance. Arms around in front of the body and palms are facing to the body (Figure 4-74). Then start with the arms from the sides of the body (Figure 4-75), rising up above the head with a deep inhale (Figure 4-76); continue with exhale while the arms coming downward in front of the center of the body (Figure 4-77) down to the level of the Dan Tian (Figure 4-78). Starting breathing naturally from this point on; hands massage along the waist to the lower back, and finger tips facing downward (Figure 4-79). Then, start to bend the body forward and downward in a motion that lengthening the spine, while use the knife edge of the hands massage along the side of the hips continue to the legs and all the way down to the feet (Figure 4-80), around the toes, end in the center (you may be able to reach the ground) (Figure 4-81), then, begin to gathering the Earth energy as the spine curving (rolling) up, starting from the lowest part of the spine to the top of the spine; loosen each spaces between the vertebras, gradually, slowly, and gently (Figure 4-82) until the upper body back to a upright position with a horse-stance, the arms in front again (Figure 4-83, 4-84 Front View). Right afterward, twist the body to your left side, stay for three seconds or a little longer (Figure 4-85) then, twist the body to your right side in a gradual and even pace, hold the posture for three seconds or a little longer (Figure 4-86), then back to the center position (Figure 4-87). Repeat the motion 3 times to 9 times.

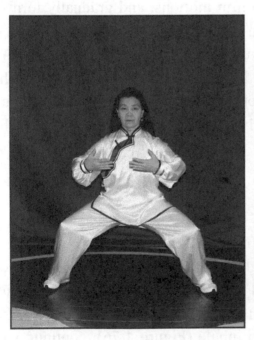
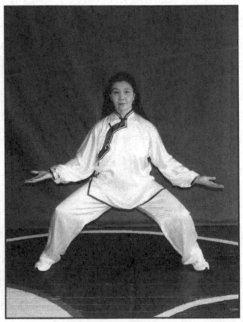

Figure 4-74   Figure 4-75

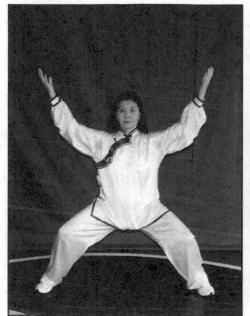

Figure 4-76

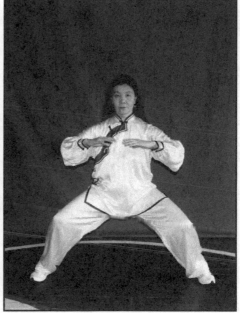

Figure 4-77

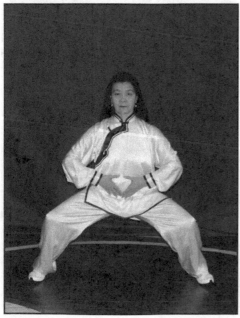

Figure 4-78

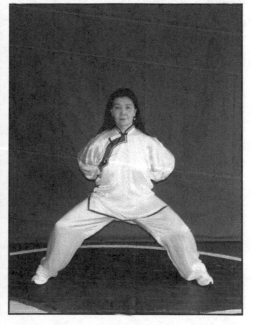

Figure 4-79

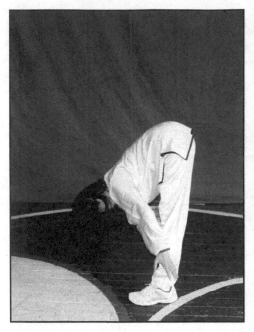

Figure 4-80

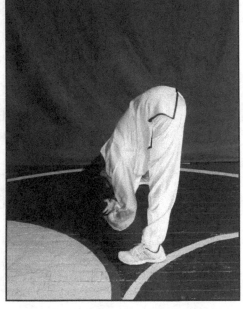

Figure 4-81

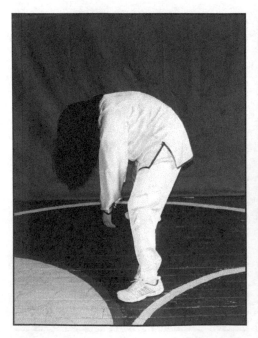

Figure 4-82

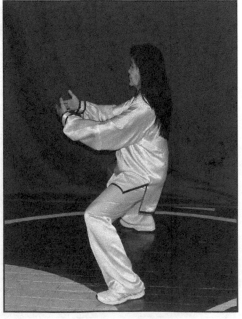

Figure 4-83 (Side View)

143

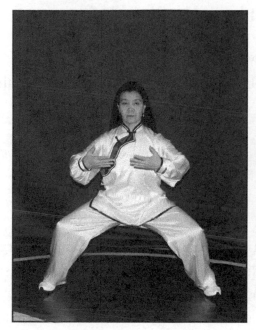
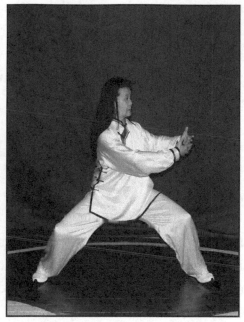

Figure 4-84 (Front View)   Figure 4-85

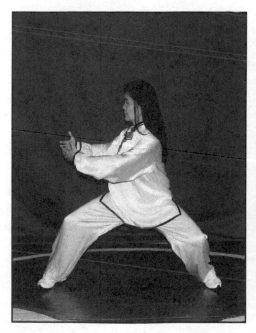
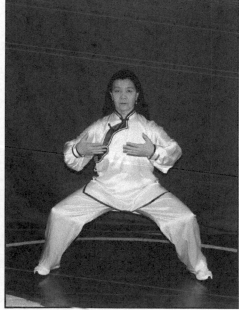

Figure 4-86   Figure 4-87

Important points on practicing the physical movements:

a. Forming a horse-stance according your own physical conditions.

b. Rolling up the spine gradually, slowly, and gently.

c. Remaining in cultivating the central spiral energy when twisting the body.

3. Nurturing the Spirit –养神

Meridian study:

The three Dan Tians is a Qi Gong term and concept of three major energy centers of the human body. No meridian channels involved. There are six points (areas) and the center of the body need to be focused on.

Health benefits: Developing into calmness through three Dan Tians meditation to nourish the spirit, the principle of conscious life, and physical functions.

Qi and The Three Dan Tians

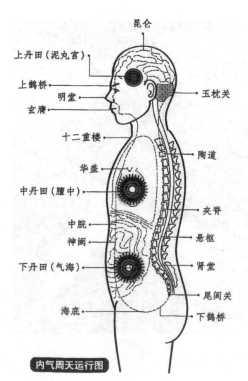

The Three Dan Tians

The Chinese classical theory of the three energy centers

Beyond physical health, Qi Gong cultivation is a mind-body integrative practice which works with a growing awareness and enhancement of the "Qi" within the body as well as surrounding the body. Qi cultivation involves a complex internal communications and interactions between the mind and the body at the spiritual, mental, energetic levels. The combination of the influences of Daoist philosophy, medicine, and martial arts made Chinese culture, and as they all recognize the theory of the three Dan Tians 丹田, it is no wonder that Dan Tian concept has been employed in these traditions for the purposes of increased energy, better health and inner balance.

Dan Tian, is written with two Chinese characters: Dan means Elixir, Tian means field. To understand the words themselves, it is said that Dan Tian is a space that something can grow from; like a seeds can grow into a flower. In medical Qi Gong practice, they are not single acupuncture points, but small areas of few acupuncture points that that Dan Tian's center location. Commonly, the phrase *Dan Tian* often refers to only the lower Dan Tian which is the area below the navel.

The three Dan Tians are areas of the body that correspond to what the ancient Daoist describe as the Three Cinnabar Fields. They were considered to be the central palaces of the body. The maintenance of freely circulating Qi through these areas was said to enable a person to have a long and healthful life. If the circulation of Qi became obstructed in the Dan Tians, disease and an early death would occur.

These three areas can also be interpreted as focal points of different physical and psychological functions of the body. Dao believers, and Qi Gong practitioners all practice energy cultivation in the three Dan Tians to establish the communications of physical and emotional energy and balancing them for health and longevity. Each of the Dan Tians is an energy area of their own, that is composed, usually, from a group of acupuncture points which are commonly used by Chinese medical practitioners.

• **The Lower Dan Tian effects and reflects the foundations of health.**

The lower Dan Tian, located in the lower abdomen between the navel and the public bone is related the acupuncture points CV4, CV5, CV6, and CV7, in which correspond to the physical functions of digestion, elimination and reproduction. Psychologically it functions as our sense of stability, balance, the nature of instinct, and as the connection to our sexuality. Daoist martial arts and Qi Gong practice pay special attention to this area as the most important center of human health and physical power.

Sinking your Qi into your lower Dan Tian is a way to begin Qi Gong practice, as well as one of the goals of practice. It is a physical requirement combined with mental achievement. When the practice gets to a good level of Qi-sinking-into-Dan Tian 气沉丹田. You have grounded your physical center, and managed a truly lowered center gravity thereby maintaining the principles of Qi Gong that support the entire practice. When the Qi can sink into the lower Dan Tian, the Dan Tian stored energy for the whole body. It also means obtaining a notable result is felt in the lungs through relaxed breathing, and an easy pace of heart beats, which help to soften the body internally and externally.

• **Middle Dan Tian is regarding the health of the emotions.**

The middle Dan Tian, is located in the center of the chest between the breasts. The related acupuncture points CV17, which corresponds to the physical functions of respiration and the circulation system of the blood and Qi. Psychologically, the middle Dan Tian functions as the emotional and interaction center of the body.

This is the balance control for emotional health. In TCM, the Lung meridian which is related to the middle Dan Tian, opening the heart and deep breathing is the need for relaxation and calmness, and to prevent mental diseases.

• **Upper Dan Tian is regarding spiritual of health.**

The upper Dan Tian, is located in the center of the forehead and is related to the acupuncture point EX-HN3, which corresponds to the physical functioning of the brain and sensory organs and to the psychological processes of thinking and contemplation.

This is also sometimes called "the third eyes" in meaning of seeing with the mind and imagination. This "eye" sees further than our physical eyes can see. The head is the home of Yang energy in the body that balance to our Yin energy.

• **Relationship of the Three Dan Tians**

A good human life is about the mind, body, and spirit being engaged and strong. The close relationship of these three Dan Tians makes an united power to guide the body's energy. The lower Dan Tian supports the middle and upper Dan Tian as a root; the upper Dan Tian intellectually possesses and guide the middle and lower Dan Tian; the middle Dan Tian connects the lower and upper Dan Tian and is the result of the effect of this connection. The middle Dan Tian dominants the relationship of the other two Dan Tians because the passion of the heart knowing a true power. Each human holds his or her own power in their heart - the middle Dan Tian. The middle Dan Tian can influence and make a difference in lives of others.

Human beings are existence with mind, body, and spirit connections. The silent energy transmissions between the three Dan Tians and through their own connective channels supports the essence of life, flows the energy, and nurtures the spirit all at their own natural settings, and paced by their own treasured routines. The three Dan Tians work together to accomplish the calmness and harmony of the body that mix with the natural energy of the universe to obtain the victory of longevity.

Human beings are about interactions with other human beings. Our universal thoughts and understanding are absolutely not limited by cultures and languages. We can simply imagine that everyone is a small universe that made of Yin and Yang, which naturally invented a personal energy field that begins where one stands and his or her feet are rooted on the Earth, extending the physical distance that his or her arms and hands can reach in a rounded shape - We are all the same in this basic energetic sense.

Therefore, the personal energy field is just a self-accomplished small world, each one filled with very similar human's energy. When a personal energy is very positive and powerful, he or she can brings out these special capabilities and possibilities to transmit it to others. Especially in helping others, nothing heals like the powerful and transmissible of a healthy human energy can do.

Qi Gong Movement:
3. Nurturing the Spirit (Human 3 of 3)

This section is the last section of this set and done by a fundamental standing posture. The palms position change on each of total three levels. Practicing with meditation is optional but the silence and calmness is required.

Start in a standing posture, the palms at the height of your lower Dan Tian level with your eyes closed between 30 seconds and 3 minutes. (Figure 4-88). Feeling the natural fundamental energy of human beings - a source of Qi which began at birth. This standing posture establishes the awareness derived not from touching but feeling of the connections between your own palms and the lower Dan Tian. This is to develop an understanding of the Dan Tian, the center through sensation.

In standing posture, move the arms at the height of middle Dan Tian, palms are facing the solar plexus, or the heart; the eyes open with a gentle and soft vision, standing between 30 seconds and 3 minutes (Figure 4-89). This is to feel the middle Dan Tian and its relationship with the lower and upped Dan Tians. More important, is to open the heart in a gentle way. Since the middle Dan Tian effects the wellness of the lower and upper Dan Tians, this can be a long process of building a closer relationship between the three Dan Tians .

Moving onto the next with the same standing posture, arms are moving upward reaching the height of the upper Dan Tian, eyes are brightly open and hold the posture between 30 seconds and 3 minutes (Figure 4-90). When the hands move upward to or a little above the head level while opening the eyes and looking far away; you will see a brighter and wider world with your own naked eyes, as well as to see a clearer inner side of yourself. The world is no longer small, the mind is no longer narrow, and stronger energy will be transferred and stored into the lower Dan Tian. The harmony of the power of the three Dan Tians makes a human body as a whole; as long as you truly understanding "The ONE," there is not much else that needs to be looked at.

In this section of cultivating energy of the three Dan Tians, the palms naturally face to yourself, arms are moving upward from narrow to wider position and from closer to the body to further from body in distance. When finish the third position, lower down the arms (Figure 4-91).

The closing of the three treasures Qi Gong, is cooling down by taking deep breaths. Arms up to breath in (Figure 4-92 and 4-93); arms down to breath out, repeat 3 times. (Figure 4-94 and 4-95), and return to a nature position (Figure 4-96).

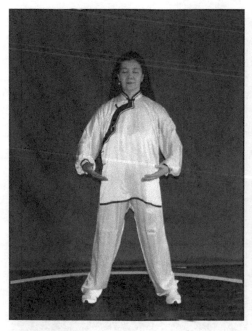

Figure 4-88

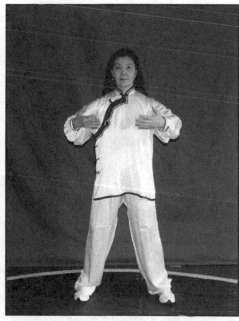

Figure 4-89

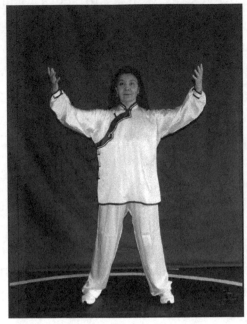

Figure 4-90

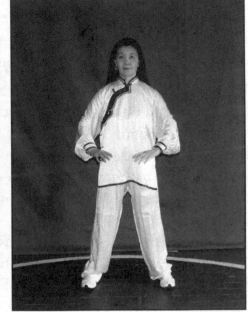

Figure 4-91

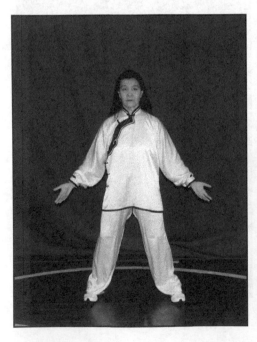

Figure 4-92

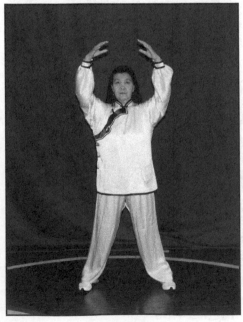

Figure 4-93

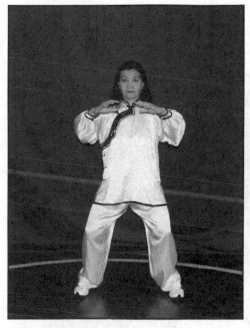

Figure 4-94

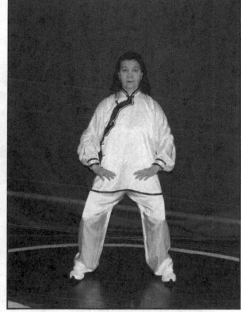

Figure 4-95

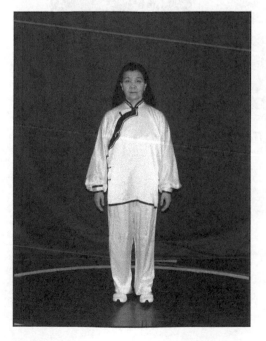

Figure 4-96

Important points on practicing the physical movements:
a. Stay centered all the time.
b. Practice in your own pace and meditate if you can.

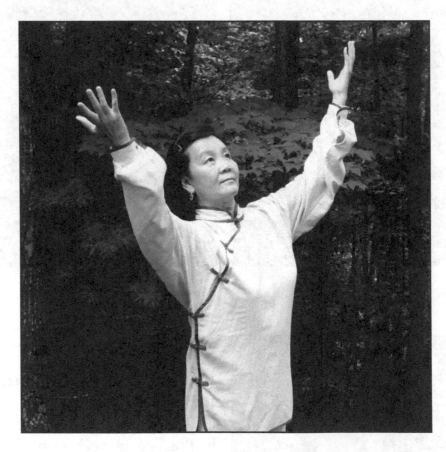

Tina Chunna Zhang practices The Three Treasures

Chapter 5

Practical Techniques in Medical Qi Gong Practice

Techniques are tools to be correctly used for manifesting principles in practice.

Healthy Breathing:

Breathing is a natural function of the human body. It is the first thing a person does when he or she is born. To some extent, people are often not aware of how they breathe, they just simply live! That is right, but, when you pay attention to how you breathe in each inhale and exhale in Qi Gong practice, you will find a better way to regulate, and improve your respiratory system.

In Qi Gong practice, we value proper breathing as one of the three primary foundations of Qi Gong along with the intension and motion.

Breathe naturally through the nose, not the mouth.

Our respiratory system is from the nose to the lungs. The lungs are a primary source of our energy level. They extract oxygen from the air we breathe, primarily on the inhale. Since the nostrils are smaller than the mouth, air exhaled through the nose creates a back pressure when one exhales. This slows the escape of air so that the lungs have more time to extract oxygen from each breath. When we breathe with the nose, the nostrils and sinuses filter warm the air into the lungs. Each nostril independently functions in filtering, warming, moisturizing, and dehumidifying the air before it goes into the lungs. Each nostril is innervated by five cranial nerves from different sides of the brain. That is how we smell the air when inhaling.

When we breathe with the mouth, there are some negative effects, such as, the mouth having no filter. Obviously breathing through the mouth is not an efficient method of breathing, especially, when exercising, or practicing Qi Gong, as mouth breathing accelerates water loss increasing the possibility dehydration, more over, makes the difficulty to breathe in lower abdomen - the Dan Tian area. This is due to mouth breathing tending to tense the muscles of the chest. Breathing through the nose limits air intake in a natural way, that eases one to slow down and keep clam. One of the benefits of proper nose breathing that Qi Gong practitioners get is reduced hypertension and lowered stress.

We also all know the nose is responsible for smelling. Smelling is a very important sensational pleasure for enjoying life, sometimes, it is for safety, too. Using the nose for each single breath is a way to maintain a keen sense of smell. Think of all the beautiful smells we take in with our nose and how smell influences our behavior and our memories through our autonomic nervous system. Sense of smell is part of our biological system that creates a branch of our conscious awareness. In Chinese culture and medicine, this essential sense is viewed as one of the abilities to help the healing process through our basic instinct response to smelling, which effects our emotions, too.

However, we can live for a while without food or water, but never without air.　Qi Gong practice is designed to exercise the diaphragm muscle and expand the lungs in a gentle way. In Chinese, we call it Tiao Xi 调息, adjust the breathing, or regulate the breathing.　There are different ways of breathing taught in different schools of Qi Gong to serve different purposes; such as: Dan Tian breathing and reversed breathing.　In medical Qi Gong, we breathe naturally.　A deep, 深, even, 均, fine, 细 and long, 长, breath is to maintain calmness, reduce an accelerated heart rate, thereby help to lower blood pressure, and regulate the level of blood sugars.

Natural breathing against holding or forcing the breathe.

When you are healthy and calm, you can breathe easily.　Without thinking about your breath, you are making an innate impulse to support your lungs and body. Each breath that you take in is receiving everything from the nature directly; each breath you breathe out is cleaning the waste in your body and getting ready for new fresh air in exchange. The body has the natural intuitive manners to breathe differently according the mood you are in at different moments. In other words, emotions effect breathing naturally.　All we can practice is to use gentle breathing to balance the emotional breathing, let the lungs help the heart.　Indeed, a deep breathing makes it possible to figure out situations and see a clearer view with new opportunities. Never hold or force your breath. Breathe naturally, like the way of breathing in your deep sleep.

Since the Qi Gong practice is a natural approach to a healthier life, listening to instinctive feelings that lead to natural opinions is also a principle. Every individual's bodily system and personal health is different and therefore their pace of breathing is different. Since the natural ways of doing things are the primary principles, there is no exceptions in breathing practice. Any forced or being controlled or unnatural breathing should absolutely be avoided.

When practicing Qi Gong breathing, you can simply close your eyes, and open your heart. Focusing your attention on your lungs, diaphragm, and lower Dan Tian areas, as if these are the only things that exist at the moment. Feel the pleasure of the lungs when they expand and enjoy every inhale and exhale, in which fulfill the biggest need and joy of a human - that is, simply to breathe. Besides breathe consciously natural and deep, you may be able to increase the feeling of the compression and expansion of the lungs, as well as diaphragm muscle, that will give you an extremely happy reason for just simply to be alive! Indeed, each breathing is appreciation to life! So, let the healthy breathing become to one of meditative ways to company your loving, passionate life!

Gentle Motion:
    "When a man is living, he is soft and supple. When he is dead, he becomes hard and rigid. When a plant is living, it is soft and tender. When it is dead, it becomes withered and dry. Hence, the hard and rigid belongs to the company of the dead; the soft and supple belong to the company of the living." - Dao De Jing

Medical Qi Gong is about using the motion to move the Qi and using the Qi to strengthen the health. The most effective way of cultivating energy and waking the nervous system is the soft and lengthening motions.

The human body is a physical gift, an indivisible entity that came with such an aggregate of features and traits; there is absolutely no exactly the same way for the variety of body types to move in the same manners, except by moving within the same set of principles. Looseness of the muscles, compression and expansion of the joints, softness of the transitional movements between each posture are the way of Qi Gong motion should be. Of course, the fundamental alignments must be learned correctly first. The preciseness of the postures must be adjudged by the body shape and physical abilities of each person. In Chinese Medical Qi Gong practice, the balance is judged in an accordance to each individual's personal limitations; anything that over doing those limitations or doing less than that person's capabilities is considered out of balance. What more important is, over doing as pushing beyond that person's physical ability can harm their original Qi.

Since this medical Qi Gong is based on meridian theory, each section has something to do with some of the energy pathways in the body. So, the practice always has to be focused on the meridians that you are strengthening and body's systems are working on, but never limited your thoughts and overlook principles like the unity of the motion. Also never forget that the meridians do not separately exist, each of them is a part of the network that makes up a system.

We are building up soft yet strong Qi Gong movements externally, that help the internal Qi flow freely in the organs and systems, that enables the organs wake up and be able to work at the their maximum efficiency. To be practically able to manage these gentle motions, you have to first overcomes any disturbance from your surroundings and any internal conflicts. When your heart is at peace, then, the gentle motions will naturally follow, and continue to help develop your balanced Qi. The healing processing will not start until the Qi can easily flow through the entire bodily system, and awareness of your own individuality reaches a higher level.

Gentle movement is a way to exercise the whole body in a specific way that has a lot to do with our joints. The joints are the most easily damaged parts of the body when people are aging. Beneath the skin, your joints are an intricate architecture of tendons, ligaments, nerves, and bones. Each of these structures is vulnerable to damage from illness or injury. If your joints hurt, even simple tasks can become a painful ordeal. The causes for the joint pain vary, but arthritis is the most common disease among them. According to "The Health Beat," a Harvard Medical School Magazine's June 2011 issue, arthritis affects one in five American adults. It is such a sad fact that high numbers of Americans have few choices except taking the pills to relieve their daily painful symptoms. It is also sad that many people believe their joint problems are simply a natural part of growing old and do not notice that plenty people age well without much arthritis. So, let's work on something you have never done and move in a way that your joints have never exercised before.

Every movement your body makes puts different kinds of pressures on your joints. Over time this wear and tear can lead to discomfort, inflammation, and sometimes more serious issues. Your joints age over time, like the rest of your body, they require comfort and support. Unfortunately, there are not many options for effective relief of pain in the joints, or programs of long term support of joint health. However, the health of your joints should not depend on how the formula based medicine is worked, either Chinese or Western. These amazing joints that we rely on every day of our lives deserve a much better care and exercise to maintain their natural abilities.

Gentle movements are a healthy supplement to support the health of the joints and one of the significant techniques of Qi Gong exercise. Remarkably, one of the foundation principles of movement in Qi Gong practice happens to make our joints healthier. The expansion and compressing of the joints in the gentle yet slow manner of Qi Gong exercises supports the over all health of the joints of the skeletal system.

Through the proper motions of Qi Gong, practitioners increase the spaces and flexibility of their joints. These movements consist of soft and open motions powered by flow, not muscular strength. When the motion around the joints or between the joints can open and expand, the energy circulation within the tendons and ligaments will be increased, more Qi will flow around all the connecting tissues which will help the joints restore whatever ability of motion they have lost. It is my belief that the joints are a really strange part of the body in that, if you don't use them, you simply lose the ability of them.

When one begins a practice of medical Qi Gong, the shoulders and hips joints normally are the stiffest. Also, the shoulders and hips joints are the biggest and most dominate joints in the body and affect every motion. Keeping loosening these joints is to increase the range of full body motion. In any movements, the smaller joints in the body are just important as the bigger joints, they must be exercised equally, otherwise, the practice is very limited; it's hard to realize these desirable and beneficial results in the fight against joints diseases and injuries. We want to get results!

When one's physical motion goes beyond one's comfort zone in practice, there is a question of control and how much further the spaces between, or around the joints can create through the lengthening? In the traditional Qi Gong practice, there is a good Chinese saying: "过犹不及," "Going too far and not going far enough are equally bad!" You should stay in a range of motion in which you feel a little beyond your physical comfort zone but haven't reached the stage of suffering pain. The range of motion, openings of the joints can only be gradually attained, along the practice level goes deeper in both physical and mindful. There are no short cuts on the way to the lifelong benefits of Qi Gong practice.

Relaxed Concentration

An old Chinese proverb says: "To nurture one's life and health, is mainly accomplished by cultivating one's mind; if the mind is calm and clear, the spirit is in a pure and healthy world; if the spirit is in a healthy world, how can illness enter you?"

The beauty of medical Qi Gong practice is its uniquely developed higher state of mind with concentration yet with relaxation. When practicing Qi Gong, the mind leads in meditative state; because the breathing and motions are gentle, even, and enjoyable, which leaves very little space for the mind to think about anything else, which helps the mind to concentrate.

Many times false things come in life because human's intellectual focus or concentration are unstable. Part of the practice of Qi Gong is practicing the ability to direct one's thinking in whatever direction one intends. Sometimes focusing on the physical movements and sometimes focusing on the calmness of the mind; either way you are working on the goal of maintaining focus, not giving in to any distractions by concentrating on what you are physically doing and what are the feelings inside you. Throughout Qi Gong practice, the mind moves with the Qi Gong movements, coordinating the mind in a relaxed manner, that will create good habits of focusing during practice; there is no judging, no competition, no separating the mind from the body; you are only aware of the joy of the whole experience. Qi Gong form exercise is highly involved in mind training exercises that also build new relationships between the body and the mind. Through many repetition of these slow yet focused exercises with Qi flowing throughout the meridian channels, a calming mind can be achieved, and the calmness of the mind develops a great focus which enables us to look at ourselves from the inside, and find our central stillness and clearness that lead to a positive way of thinking, realizing, acceptance, and control of life's balance. Physically, if the mind is calm, it can clearly feel and be very aware about what's going on, in order to prevent a sickness, or catch any illness in a very early stage and to be taken care of immediately with more and better choices for the treatments.

The mind practice in Qi Gong is a realization and examination to life. It's like taking more breaks to let the brain or mind rest from anything you do in your every busy day. This will make you realize how busy your mind is, even on your weekend or vacations! Too much activeness creates a kind of tension over time, a tensed mind needs to rest to maintain its energy flow. For instance: one of the goals in the standing practices that all Qi Gong practitioners do is to clear and empty the mind of thoughts. In the beginning, this quiet time may bring up a lot of thoughts and emotions. Try to fade them out little by little, and ignore any disturbance from your surroundings, no matter what they are. For many people, it is not so easy to be calm inside of their mind, but just like other things in life, if you work constantly, you'll harvest from the seeds you originally plant.

Relaxing is the base for concentration and clarity. It's hard to concentrate on doing something, or focus on achievements without relaxation, and the effective intellectual activity that takes place in the brain mainly requires clarity. When Qi calmly flowing through the entire body including the brain will give the mind a break to slow it down and deliver manageable thought, and these clear senses of self and mindful feelings about self, overcome disturbances, and relax the mind, allowing it to focus. When the practice has reached a higher level that is not only about physical abilities, but about qualities of understanding at the profound, relaxed, stillness stage of the mind, the noble art of healing will start. Increasing the power of the mind can control everything in the universe, and most problems have solutions because the mind can find them!

Relaxing the mind is fundamental in Qi Gong practice. In these practices the mind explores the entering of tranquility and discovers the pleasures and joy of emptiness or nothingness, yet this is not the immediate goal to achieve. First is the beginning of practicing sorting what's worth keeping in life, and what one should not carry around all the time. This will keep one's moods under control, and free from mental illnesses caused by anxiety, fear, pain, depression, and to appreciate what you have and to love who you are. Even though, the relaxing of the mind still limits the mind in a "feeling better" stage, the farther the journey goes the mind becomes elevated in a relatively permanent state where peace and satisfaction would be as natural and functional as living in your own comfortable home. However, relaxing the mind is a tool bring one's focus, into the mental realm of inner peace and clarity; the clarity of the mind is a health stage in which creativity plays, which leads to greater happiness in life experience.

When the mind calm, the body is synchronized with the Qi, and harmonized with the movements naturally yet peacefully. The healthy breathing, gentle motion, and relaxed concentration are three significant essentials in medical Qi Gong practice; one should practice with these three main-points as a unite at the same time, and all the time. The relaxed mind comforts the body and calms the breathing; the deep breathing softens the body and eases the mind; the soft body motion energizes the mind and regulates the breathing. These three blended techniques transfer the details of practice, and complementing to each other to expand into a powerful skill for a healthier and more peaceful life.

Beside daily Qi Gong practice, one should also nurture the mind with healthy food and water to give nutrition to support the physical functions and activities of our brain and mind that wishes, dreams, and creates!

Invisible Needles

Invisible needles protect you from invisible enemies!

One of the purposes of acupuncture treatment is to releases pain and helps break through the energy blockage in the meridian channels; Qi Gong exercises can do the same, perhaps even better.

Visible acupuncture needles when used to accurately puncture into the cardinal points that generate, or stimulate the positive energy to release blockages along the meridian path ways. This is a major sharing of fundamental theory between the acupuncture and medical Qi Gong practice. However, acupuncture, Tui Na, or acupressure massage are widely accepted by people as belonging to the category of the treatment, which someone else to help you. Qi Gong is a practice by oneself or a group of people with a great deal of self-correction of the postures and alignments according to the principles with a serious study, that will become to a real help to personal health. You'll gradually get to understand your health through a way of your own consciousness. Besides, the daily practice doesn't require any equipment or other's help, no appointments are necessary and you can "doctor" yourself every day.

Comparing the treatments of acupuncture or massage and medical Qi Gong, they serve the health in one common purpose - that they will help to release the tension and energy blockages. The advantage of Qi Gong practice compare to the treatment is, one knows their own uncomfortable areas and symptoms logically better than other people will. Hands - on treatments are not always available but you are the one always there to treat yourself. To be able to practice Qi Gong to serve medically, one must keep in mind, that in each section of the medical Qi Gong form is practiced to circulate Qi in the meridians, increase the flow of Qi through the meridians to maintain good health. A healthier person, is who do not give a chance to the pain or illness, or defend the cause of ill successfully through his or her stronger immune system. In addition, instead of acupuncture treatments that sometimes are limited to local areas or specific meridians, Qi Gong practice is a positive energy with motion that always working on the whole body through all the meridians. Furthermore, we are not putting treatments as a first goal; maintaining an excellent health is the treatment for a long healthy life.

Commonly, some of the popularly used acupuncture point areas in your body will be more responsive than other areas of the body when you practice. Some meridian channels are more sensitive within you than the other channels that you can feel. You should let your focus go toward these specific areas of your body that are around the one or a few acupuncture points when you practice instead of focusing on a needle sized point. For exsaple: if you have lower back pain, focus on that area and select some of the Qi Gong movements to exercise that area to reduce the uncomfortable symptoms. This is exactly like one of the traditions in acupuncture practice addressed: "The needle goes into where the pain is located." When you awaken the inner energy of your own body with a knowledge of meridian theory, each section of the Qi Gong practice eventually will become a deeper discovering of your own body and mind. In truth, medical Qi Gong practice will be like using the "invisible" needles to stimulate the points on the Qi channels, cultivates a good level of Qi and balances one's life.

Chapter 6

The Harmony of Human and Nature

"Heaven lasts long, and earth abides. What is the secret of their durability? Is it not because they do not live for themselves that they can live so long"? - Dao De Jing

"The wise take delight in water, the benevolent in mountains. The wise are active, while the benevolent are still. The wise enjoy life, while the benevolent achieve longevity." - Zhuang Zi.

Living a Harmonious Life in Three Treasured Steps:

Human life and all natural life, exists only because of the existence of the Heaven and Earth, who extend their own existence to all living things. Their Yin and Yang nature creates human life and gives the power to people to go far beyond their given biological functions, and can expanded their physical gifts into intellectual innovations. However, the living elements of the universe, such as mountains, trees, rivers and animals are also composed of and nurtured by Heaven and Earth. The basic sharing of all living things on this planet has to be harmonized, and we all need to help each other to make a calm, peaceful and productive world.

Human beings create much of their own wonderful world and enjoy most of their lives. People also live with their problems and working on them to bring the best solutions as they can. The flow of innate nature should be a basic philosophy and way of looking at life, that can be raised from the intellect or the constitution of the mind. Enjoying living should be the first priority of people's lives, not alway only pursuing their material dreams. Fortunately, each person is born to be good at something that helps keep the world naturally balanced, and any extra wishes or actions will throw off the person's natural balance and become harmful to their life.

Life is a wonderful and valuable gift that we are given from the Heaven and Earth. We create something each day to celebrate the happiness of existing; we make some dreams come true each day with our passions; we each in our own way change the world a bit.

To be able to let every person live happily on the planet, they must be passionate for something, this is the key to having a successful happy life. If you don't have any passion for anything, you don't have energy to do anything. No matter how instantly you get some expert's advise or inspiration through lectures or retreats, sometimes, you only get temporarily motivated and so easily go back to your old way of thinking and doing things. Success and happiness both are the dreams of life, they emerge into one prettier view when it's in a bigger picture: your thinking should not be limited in looking at financial success as the only way to prove your are a successful person, instead of realizing that anything you love to gain, regardless big or small, they are all will raise your spirits, they are all your successes. You can be successful in doing anything as long as your goals are achieved, and satisfaction is attained as a result of doing the things you are passionate about, It is just as simple as that! However, motivation, energy, and not giving up are the essentials on the path to success. Passion in the heart is the generator which transfers thoughts into every action that builds strong character, the qualities of honesty, and courage; that come along on the true path of success. In a life experience, the most important thing is not how talented you are but how passionately you are into something that interested you and never giving up. A passion is a powerful emotion that encourage you all the time and make you cannot wait to do the things you love to do. It's very possible that everybody has some feelings like that in certain degrees, keep going until you success. If you don't have any feeling or action like that, keep looking for what you really want in life! You cannot be happy or successful without any passion for something in your heart!

It may help to live a dreamed life with each person's nature if we truly understand the quote of Steve Jobs: "Your time is limited, so don't waste it living someone else's life. Don't be trapped by dogma, which is living with the results of other people's thinking. Don't let the noise of other's opinions drown out your own inner voice; and most important, have the courage to follow your heart and intuition. They somehow already know what you truly want to become. Everything else is secondary." A genius's exceptional capacity is a lot to with his extraordinary focus!

Life, happiness, and success should be simple. There is no need to make a great thing complicated. Here are a few famous legendary philosophical stories from Chinese history that may wake you up, make you ready to take these simple three steps for a happier and more successful life!

1. Believe in yourself:

Beliefs create a natural confidence about who you are and about defining yourself by yourself. Beliefs are the foundation of one's happiness.

This is a story that may be too childish for you, but a pure young heart may be the only thing that you lack...

A little mouse wanted to live as one of the best and most intelligent beings in the world. He heard that the sky is the most powerful thing in the universe because nothing is above it. He went to the sky to ask to be as powerful as the sky. The sky said that he was not the most powerful one because the cloud can block him from seeing below. The little mouse immediately turned to the cloud to ask how to learn to be powerful. The cloud did not think he was the most powerful one since the wind can blow him away. The little mouse suddenly thought about what the cloud said and thought it would be a great idea to see the wind and learn from him. The wind referred the little mouse to the wall because the wall is the one who could block the wind easily. When the little mouse met the wall, the wall claimed himself to be the one who had the most power, but one thing he always worried about was the fear of a hole that a mouse dug in him might become bigger and bigger and eventually make the wall fall down. Now, the little mouse thought this over and over and realized that he himself was a power being!

Everyone is an unparalleled individual, instead of traveling and seeking guidance or trying to be someone else, it's better just be yourself and understand yourself. No matter who you were in the past, you are who you are now, and who you will be growing into. On the beautiful path of life, often remind yourself that it takes a lot of time and effort to accomplish anything, sometimes, even just one thing. There is no secret rather than staying strong and persistently being real yourself.

Believing in yourself is an essential and absolutely necessary for success and a fundamental that makes nothing impossible!

2. Positive Thoughts

Once upon time, a hard working scholar was going to take an important examination that would give him a unique possibility to have a job in the royal palace if he passed the exam. The day before the examination, when he woke up in the morning, he remembered nothing but three dreams he had at the night. The first dream was that he planted vegetables on the roof of a house; the second dream was that he wore a grass-made-hat and with an umbrella walking in the rain; the third dream was that he had slept with a women he loved in back to back position. These dreams made him worry about if the dreams were a good or bad sign for the exam. So, he went to the fortune teller to get advice. The fortune teller's answer to the dreams were negative as: the first dream meant that the scholar will fail the exam because it makes no sense to grow vegetables on the roof of a house; the second dream meant that as it was unnecessary to have a hat and an umbrella because that only duplicate things, there was no logical in that dream either; his third dream totally killed any chance of success as it was a laughable way for lovers to sleep together. The negative result from this fortune teller was that it was simply impossible for him to pass the exam, he'd better to give up, and go home.

He thought about how hard he had been worked to prepare for the exam, and if he got the job, he could feed not only his starving family but maybe the whole village he lived. He could not believe that was the end of his longing for that job. So, he went to a different fortune teller for an answer. The second fortune teller's answers were positive: The first dream was a sign of unique way to grow vegetable by getting a closer distance to the Sun light than the plant that were growing on the ground; the second dream's result was double protection on a rainy day; and the third dream just meant that it would be a turning point obtained by turning the position towards the women he loved.

Of course, he passed the exam, and a dream came true!

Many times in life, what looks big is usually small; what looks scary usually has a joyful side, what seems impossible may be a very much achievable. Everything comes from one's inside thoughts. For instance, being happy doesn't mean that everything in life is perfect, it means that you've decided to look beyond the imperfections, and accept your own imperfections as well as other people's imperfections. In matter of fact, in everyone's life, there is always someone better than you, some things you will never have. Even if you are the best fighter, there are the fights you don't win! If you understand this from the heart, not from the words, you may always be prepared to accept the negativities with a positive attitude, take everything easy, look at the bigger picture. Setting healthy as your first priority, meanwhile, positive thinking helps one avoid emotional suffering. Positive reactions balance the mind, which should please you by allowing yourself to express your true feelings and react with your natural instinctual emotions. Positive thinking also enable you to adjust and release negativities soon enough that they will not hurt you bad enough to disturb your emotional balance, or injure you bad enough to lead to any physical abnormalities. Positive thinking is the groundwork that happiness builds on.

As a Chinese proverb says, " An easily satisfied person is the one who will be forever happy." Happiness is a state of mind where you are temporarily satisfied with what you do and what you have at that moment. Life events may change happiness from time to time. When worse things happen, even a generally happy person may have sad days. However, a real happy person is the one who has a positive attitude about life and is confident in his or her town identity. Taking a good life philosophy is a tool or guidance to a person's satisfaction. As one of Chinese proverbs says: "Satisfaction limits anger, and extends age."

The world and things in life really depend on how you look at them. Thoughts and view points make a person who would be a positive or negative one, happy or unhappy one. It is not about what has happened in life, because something is always happening, it is how you react to what's happening.

3. It's all about Freedom

"A path is formed because we walk on it; a thing has a name because we call it so." - Zhuang Zi.

"The highest achievement of the Dao, is freedom of the soul." - Tina Chunna Zhang

Living free is living with liberated thoughts, no matter who you are and what you are doing, free yourself from the limitations, following the nature of your soul that the Heaven and Earth has created, in which, the natural state of mind will fulfill your joy!

Freedom is simplicity

Being simple is a quality.

We all were born naked and we cannot carry anything with us when leaving this world, everything is a passing by of life, so why do we spend a large amount of our life time chasing unnecessary things?

The world changes and technology develops to make our life easier and more enjoyable. In this materialistically overwhelming world, many people easily fall into a burning desire to chase the best materials without considering their own abilities. Their lives become trapped into a race with no apparent final destination. This cost so much time and energy in exchange for these result of discovering: there is always someone who is better than you, there is somethings that you never be able to have, there is someone you cannot be - these are to say, that your heart of freedom is totally lost. To be able to establish the real value of materials, the idea of "Enough" could be the perfect thought to stop the chasing the unnecessaries, starting enjoying what you have, and spending time and energy on someone you love, something you are passionate for, and realize some dreams in your ordinary yet special life that you don't want to regret when you leave this world permanently.

If a life is based on a simplicity, one can understand themselves better and look at things from a higher position without being disturbed much   Looking closely at the quality of everything becomes more important, eventually, the material become items which you are no longer interested in unless you need them. You will be no longer tempted because your mind now has perfect judgment, which everything's value is careful ascertained before selection.

Freedom as a path

Freedom is a path that we walk on freely.

Between the Heaven and Earth, there was no indication of the directions of east, west, north and south, as the directions existed long after nature came into being. There was no beliefs until we believed them. We find somewhere to walk and then, it becomes a path that many people will walk on.

The brain doesn't pay attention to boring things, It likes to be charged by attractive things, new things and changes. Being creative is not easy, because some people have the minds of a slave and their thoughts are not free. For example, we see people or friends who seems to understand and speak beautifully about wisdom and freedom, but cannot make any effort to apply that knowledge or ideas to their own lives. Their lives are still full of complaints about many things. This is because their intellectual knowledge is still not a knowledge that becomes a real life path that leads to the freedom of the mind. The ability of the mind that creates new thoughts is based on freedom of the imagination, which   transcends traditional ideas, imaginations, patterns, etc. to form new ideas, methods, inventions, and life changes. Without freedom, the mind can only work by rules and limitations.

The freedom also gives thoughts plenty of space and power to think things over and over, clearly and carefully focus on what it is. Especially on the new ideas that will become either a creative product or outstanding piece of art work. The freedom of the energy will be directed by free thinking, with full passion that leads to the excellence – the major step onto the path of any kind of successes.

When people really walk on the path of freedom, their new dreams come true and success follows, there are no limitations.

Freedom is flow

Water seeks its own level.

Every individual has their own heart of freedom, and their own usual, normal, characteristic selves. Through many ups and downs in life, they are themselves and keep changing harmoniously with nature.

It is not possible or necessary that each one of us needs to be, or can be, on the same level of success. Life is a mystery that some people surely know better than others; and life is always unequal. Expect some unfairness is a practical art. Everyone has their own uniqueness and talented on something, that makes each life following their own rhythm and flow, in which one can find their potentials, realize their dreams. Instead of struggling with trying to win all the games in life, one should wisely chose to engage and pursue the possibilities, that can practically make the ordinary into the extraordinary within one's standards.

Water seeks its own level and naturally flows. Freedom is the same. Freedom cannot be formulated or forced; it's all about how far the mind can go. It sets a positive attitude to look at the world and life, it builds the fundamentals of happiness, it brings a flow like water nurtures the thoughts. The freedom of the mind creates the freedom of one's physical energy and the appearance of someone whom others enjoy being around. One who has a free soul can inspire other people, they are also the character of stimulating, uplifting, easy going and with an acceptance of all styles of life and are not afraid to leave their own comfort zone.

Freedom is a way of independence, too. That sets one free from negative attachments in mind, and declares your freedom from the past, freedom from insecurity, freedom from fear, and freedom from anything and anyone holding you back from being the individual you created to be!

Freedom is in the heart. No matter how free a person can be, he or she still has some limited states of mind and negative manners from time to time. You cannot win all the fights, but you can regain freedom and stand up after being knocked down, continue to fight for freedom. However, part of the flow of a life with freedom is to perceive the meaning of "falling down is part of life, and getting back up is living!" We do not expect the freedom is always there, even it should be a natural part of human nature, it is like everything else, we have to work to achieve.

In addition, the level of freedom of the minds are varied depend on the education and experiences of each individual, how they reflect and respond to the world around them, and how they adopt which principles of living. As long as people can free themselves from the prisons of their past failures and make room for something new, they can always regain freedom of the soul. Then, they will have more flow in their lives regardless of the situation they live in, rich or poor.

Since the Dao is impossible to define precisely, it only can be discovered through our own nature and experience; each human's nature is ever changing as well as always the same. There is never a conclusion but forever the possibilities and new discoveries of living free!

The Yellow Emperor's Classic of Internal Medicine

《黃帝内经》：上古天真论篇第一

昔在黃帝，生而神靈，弱而能言，幼而徇齊，長而敦敏，成而登天。乃問於天師曰：余聞上古之人，春秋皆度百歲，而動作不衰；今時之人，年半百而動作皆衰者，時世異耶，人將失之耶。岐伯對曰：上古之人，其知道者，法於陰陽，和於術數，食飲有節，起居有常，不妄作勞，故能形與神俱，而盡終其天年，度百歲乃去。今時之人不然也，以酒為漿，以妄為常，醉以入房，以欲竭其精，以耗散其真，不知持滿，不時御神，務快其心，逆於生樂，起居無節，故半百而衰也。

夫上古聖人之教下也，皆謂之虛邪賊風，避之有時，恬淡虛無，真氣從之，精神內守，病安從來。是以志閒而少欲，心安而不懼，形勞而不倦，氣從以順，各從其欲，皆得所願。故美其食，任其服，樂其俗，高下不相慕，其民故曰朴。是以嗜欲不能勞其目，淫邪不能惑其心，愚智賢不肖不懼於物，故合於道。所以能年皆度百歲，而動作不衰者，以其德全不危也。

帝曰：人年老而無子者，材力盡耶，將天數然也。岐伯曰：女子七歲。腎氣盛，齒更髮長；二七而天癸至，任脈通，太衝脈盛，月事以時下，故有子；三七，腎氣平均，故真牙生而長極；四七，筋骨堅，髮長極，身體盛壯；五七，陽明脈衰，面始焦，髮始墮；六七，三陽脈衰於上，面皆焦，髮始白；七七，任脈虛，太衝脈衰少，天癸竭，地道不通，故形壞而無子也。丈夫八歲，腎氣實，髮長齒更；二八，腎氣盛，天癸至，精氣溢寫，陰陽和，故能有子；三八，腎氣平均，筋骨勁強，故真牙生而長極；四八，筋骨隆盛，肌肉滿壯；五八，腎氣衰，發墮齒槁；六八，陽氣衰竭於上，面焦，髮鬢頒白；七八，肝氣衰，筋不能動，天癸竭，精少，腎藏衰，形體皆極；八八，則齒髮去。腎者主水，受五藏六府之精而藏之，故五藏盛，乃能寫。今五藏皆衰，筋骨解墮，天癸盡矣。故髮鬢白，身體重，行步不正，而無子耳。

帝曰：有其年已老而有子者何也。岐伯曰：此其天壽過度，氣脈常通，而腎氣有餘也。此雖有子，男不過盡八八，女不過盡七七，而天地之精氣皆竭矣。

帝曰：夫道者年皆百數，能有子乎。岐伯曰：夫道者能卻老而全形，身年雖壽，能生子也。

　　黃帝曰：余聞上古有真人者，提挈天地，把握陰陽，呼吸精氣，獨立守神，肌肉若一，故能壽敝天地，無有終時，此其道生。中古之時，有至人者，淳德全道，和於陰陽，調於四時，去世離俗，積精全神，遊行天地之間，視聽八達之外，此蓋益其壽命而強者也，亦歸於真人。其次有聖人者，處天地之和，從八風之理，適嗜欲於世俗之間。無恚嗔之心，行不欲離於世，被服章，舉不欲觀於俗，外不勞形於事，內無思想之患，以恬愉為務，以自得為功，形體不敝，精神不散，亦可以百數。其次有賢人者，法則天地，像似日月，辨列星辰，逆從陰陽，分別四時，將從上古合同於道，亦可使益壽而有極時。

Translation by Tina Chuuna Zhang

The Yellow Emperor's Classic of Internal Medicine

Chapter 1
On the Superior Men of Ancient Times

A long, long time ago, the Yellow Emperor was a born talent. He was very good at words and had a great capacity for thought and knowledge. Through hard, diligent study, he finally became the Emperor of China. One day, the Yellow Emperor asked his royal family doctor who's name was Qi Bo: "I have heard that people of ancient times had lived as long as over 100 years with no signs of weakening in movements, but people nowadays become weakened in their movements at the age of 50 years old. Is this because of the different in times or the way people lived?

Qi Bo answered: "The ancient people who knew the Dao, had a proper way to live. They followed the pattern of Yin and Yang, remained in harmony with numerical symbols, ate and drank with moderation and lived their daily life in a regular pattern with neither excess nor abuse. In this way, their spirits and bodies remained in perfect harmony with each other, they could live their natural life for over 100 years."

"On the other hand, people now are quite different from then. They replace their water with alcohol; consider the wild-fantasy as normal; have sexual relations while intoxicated; exhaust pure energy through useless desires and waste true energy through mindlessness and carelessness. These resulted in failing to maintain their energy and guard their spirit constantly. These cause their hearts to go opposite from their happiness, and they live their daily life in an irregular pattern. This is the reason that they can only live half of their life span."

Qi Bo continued: "The teachings of the Sages of ancient times on nurturing life was that one should avoid bad weather and unhealthy environments, living a quiet life without too many desires, so one can maintain his pure energy, and peaceful spirit, then disease cannot enter the body. Consequently, one can have a very calm heart, that is, having a peaceful mind without fear and working hard without fatigue. When the energy is flowing, one can obtain satisfaction of every need. Then, people would all be like: any food that available to them is delicious, any clothes that they wearing are beautiful. They love their culture, customs, and are pleased in the society with whatever class they belong to. These are truly simple and satisfied people. Moreover, their eyes are never attacked by unwanted luxuries; their mind won't be fooled by vicious objects; and their thoughts never focus on material gains or losses. Regardless if one is a fool or intelligent, capable or dumb, they retain their perfect virtue that won't be influenced by the temptations of the surroundings. These are the reasons people can live long since they have never been exposed to dangers, and managed to retain the excellence of virtue principles. This is the Dao of life."

The Yellow Emperor asked another question: "When a man grows older, he cannot have children. Is it because his energy has already been exhausted or because it is a natural age restriction?" Qi Bo replied: "The kidney's Qi of a woman becomes in abundance at the age of 7, her baby teeth are replaced by permanent ones, and her hair grows longer. At the age of 14, a woman's conception meridian begins to flow, her menstruation arrives, and she is capable of becoming pregnant. At the age of 21, a woman becomes adult, full of energy in her kidneys, and her last tooth begins to grow with all other teeth completed. At the age of 28, tendons and bones grow stronger, the hair grows to the longest, and the body is in the greatest conditions. At the age of 35, the brighter Yang meridians become weaker, her appearance starts to withdraw, her hair begins falling off. At the age of 42, the three Yang meridians are weaker, she looks even more withdrawn, and her hair begins turning gray. At the age of 49, the energy of the conception meridian is in deficiency, and menstruation stops. Her body shape changes and she cannot become pregnant anymore."

"As to man, his kidneys Qi becomes plentiful at the age of 8. His hair grow fuller, longer, and the teeth change. At the age of 16, his kidney's

Qi becomes stronger and sexual energy begins to arrive, he can ejaculate and capable to have children when he has intercourse with women. At the age of 24, the kidney's energy make a man have stronger tendons and bones, his teeth are completed. At the age of 32, he has fully grown all tendons, bones and muscles. At the age of 40, the kidneys energy becomes weaker, his hair begins to fall off as well as the teeth. At the age of 48, Yang energy become weaker, starting to show in the upper body, his hair begins turning gray. At the age of 56, the liver energy become weaker, the tendons become inelastic, the body begins to look old. At the age of 64, more hair and teeth fall off. The kidneys are in charge of water, and they receive energy from other organs and store it. When the other organs are energy deficient, the kidneys lack power, so the body becomes heavy, walking steps are unstable, and he cannot have children anymore."

The Yellow Emperor asked: Some people are old but they can still have children, why is that?" Qi Bo, again, replied: "This is because they have more prenatal energy than the average, and the energy of their meridians always flow to a superior kidney energy. Although they can still have children when they are old, but their age cannot be too far beyond 64 years of age in men, and 49 years of age in women. The pure energy of Heaven and Earth will be exhausted after these ages.

The Yellow Emperor came with another question: "Some Taoists Spiritual Masters lived to be over120 years, can they still have children at that age? Qi Bo replied: "These men can have children, because they keep their bodies in perfect condition."

The Yellow Emperor said: "I have heard that in early historical times, there were "Superior Men," who knew the essence of the Heaven and Earth, mastered the principle of the Yin and Yang, regulated their breath to take pure energy from the universe, kept the spirit pure, exercised the tendons, bones, and muscles to make body as a healthy whole, so their life would be as long as the existence of the Heaven and Earth. They were the Masters of the Dao."

"In the medieval times, there were "Knowing Men," who managed to live in harmony with Yin and Yang, had excellent virtue, adjusted their lives according to the changes of the four seasons, avoided disturbing opinions of their society, cultivated their energy and flowed with nature and let the development of their sense of hearing, sight of vision be unlimited, these were their ways of achieving longevity. They belong to the "Superior Men," group also.

A "Sage," was the one who lived in the normal world, followed the laws of the nature and was freed from anger and hate. They wore common clothes and acted no different from the rest of the world. However, the sages were different from the ordinary folk. They didn't labor excessively for anything; their life purpose was to enjoy happiness and inner tranquility, their achievement was self-satisfaction on what ever they do. The result of their life style was that their bodies were never wore out and their spirits were never disturbed. They absolutely lived to be over 120 years."

"There were "Great Men" who could follow the principles of Heaven and Earth and derived their life according the Sunrise and Sunset, the change of the Moon, the map of the Stars, balancing the Yin and Yang of their body's energies and respected the differences of the four seasons. They were accompanying The Dao, and following the outstanding ideas of their ancestors, by these ways, they were able to live long."

Acknowledgment

A very special thank-you to my great mentor, Dr. Kong Si Bo (1933 - 2011). You and your family's dedication of practice have made an important part of the history of Traditional Chinese Medicine since the early 1911. The knowledge that passed on from Dr. Kong will be always shared in the field of Traditional Chinese Medicine.

I am thankful for all the Chinese doctors, Qi Gong experts who I worked with in the clinics in Beijing over the years.

I cannot thank enough for the trainings under my Martial Arts Masters: Northern Wu Style Tai Ji Quan Master Li Bing Ci, and Cheng Style Ba Gua Zhang Master Liu Jing Ru.

My deepest appreciation goes to Chinese Internal Martial Arts Master, the founder and director of Wu Tang Physical Culture Association, Frank Allen, for your outstanding teachings and advices.

No words can truly express my gratitude for decades of support from the members of Wu Tang PCA and students around the world!

Thank-you, David Beard, for the photography in the book.

Love,
Tina Chuuna Zhang

About the Author

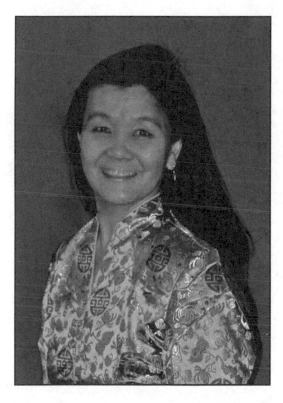

Tina Chunna Zhang is a native Chinese and moved to America in the 1980s. She experienced martial arts and Chinese folk dance throughout her childhood and youth. Through many years of study and practice Chinese Internal Martial Arts, she become the 5th generation Northern Wu Style Tai Ji Quan lineage master, and the 6th Generation Cheng Style Ba Gua Zhang lineage master.

She Studied Theory and Diagnostics at Beijing University of Traditional Chinese Medicine, and mentored privately by one of the most famous Traditional Chinese Medicine doctor Kong Si Bo (1933-2011), Beijing.

Tina is an accomplished author of Internal Martial Arts and Qi Gong books. She co-authored with Master Frank Allen the books of *"Classical Northern Wu Style Tai Ji Quan"*, and *"The Whirling Circles of Ba Gua Zhang"*. She is the program founder and author of *"Earth Qi Gong for Women"*.

Tina successfully runs a Traditional Chinese Medicine Clinic, specializing in Qi Gong treatment; and professionally teaches Qi Gong, Tai Ji Quan, and Ba Gua Zhang classes in New York City and conducts seminars worldwide.

Welcome to visit her web site at www.The3Treasures.com